D0724066

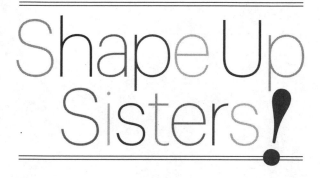

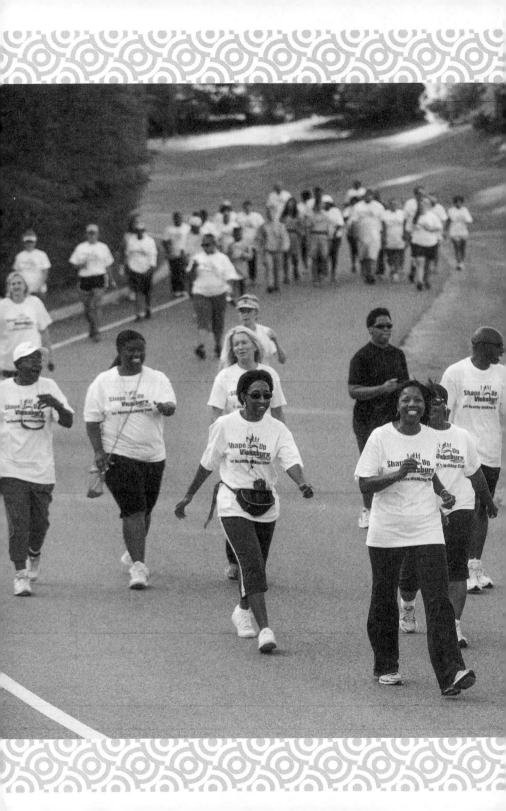

THE PERMANENT WEIGHT-LOSS AND
FITNESS PROGRAM FOR THE REST OF US

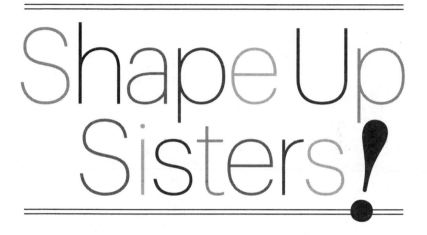

Shape Up
Sisters!

What It Took for My Town in One of America's
Fattest and Poorest States to Lose **15,000** Pounds

LINDA FONDREN

RODALE.

© 2014 by Linda Fondren

Photographs © 2014 by Rodale Inc.

Rodale books may be purchased for business or promotional use or for special sales. For information, please write to:
Special Markets Department, Rodale Inc., 733 Third Avenue, New York, NY 10017

Printed in the United States of America
Rodale Inc. makes every effort to use acid-free ♾, recycled paper ♻.

Sources for recipes on pages 203–223: National Heart, Lung, and Blood Institute; National Institutes of Health; and U.S. Department of Health and Human Services

Photographs by Mitch Mandel/Rodale Images
Book design by Joanna Williams

Library of Congress Cataloging-in-Publication Data is on file with the publisher.

ISBN 978-1-62336-144-0   paperback

Distributed to the trade by Macmillan

2   4   6   8   10   9   7   5   3   1   paperback

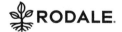

We inspire and enable people to improve their lives and the world around them.
rodalebooks.com

For my sister Mary.
We lost you too soon,
but through your death,
other women now live
without regret.

Contents

Part 3
The Shape Up Sisters Plan

Introduction

Telling It Like It Is

The battle of the bulge is a fierce one.

To win it, you need a supersize motivator like our hero Linda Fondren. Linda is a force, a sculptor, reshaping lives in Vicksburg, Mississippi. When Mississippi was named the most obese state, she got out her chisel and she went to work. She carved Shape Up Vicksburg and challenged the city to lose 17,000 pounds. She engraved healthy choices on restaurant menus and school lunches. She molded exercise classes for women and started a walking club with T-shirts that read "Walking Is Cheap, Life Is Precious."

That's what our sculptor Linda carved. All over her city. Life is precious, and so is she.

—LL Cool J, CNN Heroes presentation, 2010

F OR THE BETTER PART OF THE PAST DECADE, my home state of Mississippi had the sad distinction of topping the list of the fattest states in the nation, according to the "obesity map" put out by the Centers for Disease Control and Prevention. Mississippi is known as the Hospitality State for its charm and generosity—in fact, we're one of the top states for charitable giving—but all that Southern comfort comes with a sizable downside: Some 69 percent of our residents are overweight or downright obese. And the fact that most people in Mississippi battle the bulge is no surprise to anyone in my hometown of Vicksburg.

Vicksburg sits high on the bluff above the banks of the mighty Mississippi River, across from the Louisiana state line. It's known for blues music, Civil War history, and—like most of the South—for over-the-top obesity rates.

Because being fat is the norm here, nobody really realizes they have a problem. If the person next to you also weighs 250 pounds, then you're average, right? If what's valued is having some "meat on your bones," then why get smaller? You don't realize that fat is a sign that a lot of other things are out of whack in your life when you look like your friends, family, and neighbors.

Fat is the symptom of what our culture is feeding us. Rich or poor, black or white, fat acts the same. It creates diabetes and heart disease, fosters an environment for cancer to grow, and builds other health problems too long to list. In Mississippi, for example, more than 12 percent of adults have diabetes, according to the Trust for America's Health and the Robert Wood Johnson Foundation. Another 39 percent have high blood pressure. Our numbers might be extreme, but these are problems everywhere in America. The growing rate of obesity in our children and its deadly consequences have made weight more than just a private struggle. It's a major public health issue.

But if we collectively decide to believe that we are worth investing time and energy in, then we eat better, we start to move and enjoy our bodies, and, in this way, together, we change the culture itself. Before I tell you about what's been happening in Vicksburg to start this change, let me get a hard truth out of the way:

Most people across this county think they can't afford to lose weight.

They think they need to join a program that costs a lot of money, or they think they need their own personal trainer and private chef, like all those celebrities they see on TV. They think they need special, magical foods or supplements—gimmicks. And they just can't afford any of that.

I'm not surprised by one study that found the obesity rate among shoppers at a Seattle Whole Foods was only 4 percent, compared to 25 percent in the surrounding area. Access to fresh groceries is not the only advantage: Money affords you the ability to enroll in fancy weight-loss programs, hire that personal trainer, and even consider surgical intervention.

And then there's everybody else.

When I look around Vicksburg, I see middle- to low-income folks struggling to feed their families on a tight budget. They are more likely to buy groceries from Walmart than Whole Foods. We don't even have a Whole Foods around here. Many folks are working two jobs. Some can't find jobs at all. The unemployment rate hovers around 16 percent, and more than 32 percent of the people here live below the poverty line. Nobody has the time for involved meal planning or intricate exercise regimens. The reality is, most people I have come across in my travels around the state, as well as in other parts of the country, don't have extra money or a lot of spare time to devote to weight loss, even if they think they should.

Marketing trends keep giving us new weight-loss and exercise strategies, yet as a nation—not just here in Mississippi—we are heavier now than at any other time in our history. I believe it boils down to a disconnect between what we believe should be true and what actually is true. The messages we are getting from the media—from advertising to magazines and TV shows—are setting unrealistic goals for obese women. And few solutions attack the real issue—that dieters are being ruled by their social interactions and by beliefs and assumptions about themselves and what is possible for them. These attitudes and behaviors are setting a tone for their family and community. And so the vicious cycle continues.

When my sister died of cancer after suffering with obesity for most of her life, it caused me to really examine what I could do to help others in her situation. I realized that my own interest in fitness might be the key, so my husband and I opened a health club for women called Shape Up Sisters in Vicksburg. As you'll see in the coming chapters, I realized that in order for my clients to achieve their goals, it was going to take a shift in the way the whole town looked at food and exercise. I knew that for any weight-loss program to work on a large scale, it would need to be low-maintenance and cost-effective. I also knew we needed to use the greatest weapon we have: the ability to help each other.

So in the fall of 2009, I created a simple lifestyle program for all the residents of Vicksburg to follow for 17 weeks. I inspired City Hall to declare Shape Up Vicksburg an official city program, and I convinced local restaurants to create "Shape Up" low-calorie menu options. I created free nutrition and fitness classes that I gave at the public housing authority, at schools—at any place that would have me. The 2,500 residents who signed on to the Shape Up Vicksburg program could track their weight loss online or at weigh-in stations at Walmart and the local medical center.

During the initial sign-up meeting, people of all sizes and colors showed up. Men came and women came, many with children in tow. They had more in common than just the problem of being seriously overweight: They shared the struggle of finding work that would keep their families secure; they shared the hope for a better future; and, most of all, they shared the desire to know more about how to be healthier and eat more nutritiously.

Poverty, race, and obesity are linked together like a chain:

For the better part of this decade, Mississippi had the highest rate of obesity in the country (though the state has now been edged out by its neighbor Louisiana). Mississippi also leads the country in percentage of adults who don't exercise. (But if they gave a gold medal for porch sitting, you bet we'd be the winner.) Those people who came to the meeting, they needed more than just me, for sure, but I was the opening in a line of possibility.

After the end of the official 17-week challenge, the weight lost by hundreds of Vicksburg locals added up to a collective total of 15,000 pounds. The goal had been 17,000 pounds, so we didn't technically reach our goal. But we all still won.

The reason why: It was never about the number. It was about prompting action, getting people who felt they were too "stuck" to move. It was about coming together to help each other do more than what we could do alone. Together we accomplished more than just weight loss; we created a fundamental shift in attitude, instilling a belief that something beyond the present reality was possible. Shape Up Vicksburg became a health and fitness movement.

Today in Vicksburg, upwards of 100 people still show up every month for our free walks around city parks and through urban neighborhoods, and I have opened the gym on Saturdays, free to anyone who wants to break a sweat. Most weeks it's packed tighter than the Baptist church on Easter. In a culture that has us eating fried food, sitting on the couch, and believing that nothing is ever going to change in our lives for the better, every day I see people who want to lose weight and gain some kind of control over their health—and over their lives in general.

People around the country have wanted to know the nitty-gritty of what I started in Vicksburg. I was honored to be a CNN Hero in 2010 and have spoken to hundreds of groups, from city hall meetings to women's groups to law students at Harvard University. And I see in the letters and e-mails that flow into my office each week people always ask me the same thing: "I was so inspired by what you said. Can you tell me what to do?"

This hunger for weight-loss wisdom is what led me to write the book you're holding in your hands. What does it take to inspire an entire town to lose 15,000 pounds in a state that long held the nation's "heavyweight" title for the highest obesity rate? And how can that help you change your own life for the better? Listen up and I'll tell you.

In this book, I give you the tools to develop a determined mind-set and change your life. It's filled with daily, flexible, realistic suggestions for action and reflection, designed to integrate into your life as you live it. This is no eat-seaweed-and-do-Pilates-with-skinny-celebrities routine; it's a mind-shift prescription for real women with real problems.

This book questions the perceived norms in our communities. Norms are not simply habits but are embedded in culture and tradition. They are our attitudes and beliefs and standards we accept without question. I am passionate about reaching women and their families—where they are right now. *Shape Up Sisters!* combines all that I have learned through my life experiences; I have seen my message influence people at their cores, after peeling back the many layers of cultural and psychological norms, in a way that speaks to their hearts as well as to their minds.

In the South we use the expression "Mother Wit." The woman who's got Mother Wit has an unshakable belief in her capabilities and is clear-headed enough not to be fooled. Some of us seem to be in full possession of our Mother Wit from birth; others of us have it awakened through the school of hard knocks. Mother Wit is the essence of this book. It might be an expression that black Southern women are most likely to recognize, but I promise it speaks to all of us regardless of color or creed.

Shape Up Sisters! is built on the central message of my

gym, "Positively Reshaping Women." I've structured this book into three interlinking parts. First, I tell the story of my life and how I launched a program that inspired a whole community—and how *Shape Up Sisters!* can help you believe in your own capabilities to get the life you desire and deserve. Then, through the Mother Wit served up in the second section of this book, I'll show you how your unknown strengths are greater than your known weaknesses and perceived limitations combined. And finally, in the third section, I'll give you a practical how-to guide to nutrition and exercise built on the resources hiding right in front of you, because—here's a little secret—*you already have what you need to live healthier.*

My job is to show you how this is true so you can be inspired to cast aside the behaviors that are weighing you down, in every sense, and embrace a life filled with far better health and more possibilities. As Harriet Tubman once said, "If I could have convinced more slaves that they were slaves, I could have freed thousands more."

Now let's get to it.

Part 1
What's Behind Shape Up Sisters

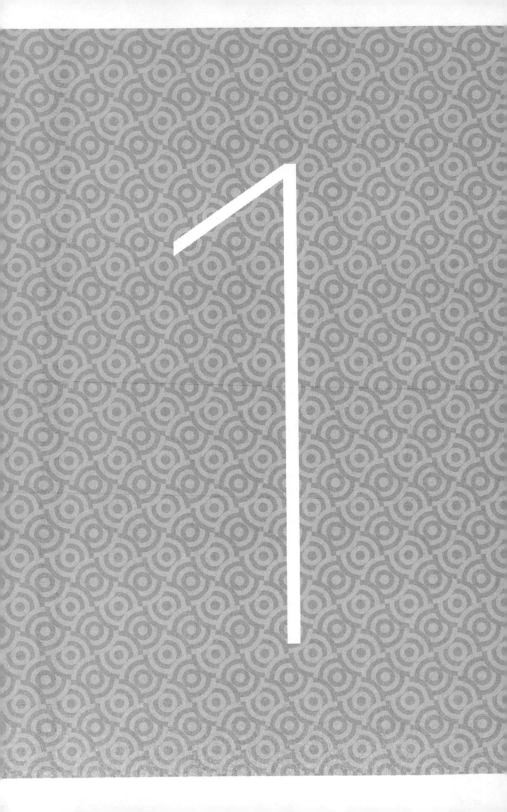

What I Came From

NO MATTER WHAT YOUR STORY HAS BEEN, you can write yourself a new one. No matter what has happened to you, your past does not define your future. No matter what choices you've made in your life, at any moment you can start making different ones. Have the drive and desire to go for it and take a chance on change, because you cannot leave the world the way you found it.

Listen to me here. I know this from personal experience.

I can't talk about my life without first talking about where and what I came from. The places you have lived can shape you as powerfully as the genes that get passed down from your family members.

Here's some background: Today, Vicksburg, Mississippi, is the seat of Warren County, 45 minutes west of Jackson, the state capital. About 23,000 people live in town and another 23,000 or so live in the surrounding area. But you can't understand

3

the place without first talking about its link to the Mississippi River and the Civil War.

A horseshoe bend in the Mississippi River gave birth to Vicksburg. It had long been a hunting and fishing ground for the native Natchez and Choctaw Indians. In 1825 it became a town, and five flags have flown from its bluff—French, Spanish, English, Confederate, and American. The combination of agriculture, the traffic from barges moving supplies up and down the river, and the railroad made it a prosperous place (it was also full of gamblers and saloons). Vicksburg is where Joseph Biedenharn bottled Coca-Cola for the first time, in 1894. It is most famous, however, for its role during the Civil War. Holding Vicksburg was the key to controlling the Mississippi River, so in 1863, she was besieged by Union forces and became a memorable chapter in history, ending the war.

I wish I could say that all was peaceful and prosperous after that, but you all know history wasn't that kind. In the late 1800s racists murdered some 50 black men in what has come to be known as the Vicksburg Massacre, and the cycle of lynching and voter suppression continued well into the civil rights era.

Today, blacks no longer belong to whites. And Vicksburg's white supremacists no longer patrol the streets with guns to convince black voters to stay home on Election Day. Yet, we still do. The jobs that left in the boom years have never really returned. Poverty and a resigned sense that "things will always be this way" make for a legacy that's hard to shake.

Mississippi has a tortured past, but it also has an evolving future. I confronted my past when I married a white man and moved back to my hometown to help make a difference. But, there are a few things you need to know first.

Comedian Steve Martin had a joke that began, "I was born a poor black child . . ." Well, in my life it was no joke. I was one of 13 children born during a time in the South when it was not okay for people who looked like me to walk through the front door of nice establishments. We lived in a series of shotgun houses, wherever we could afford rent, in different parts of Vicksburg. We were poor, plain and simple. A decent meal was hard to come by. I remember eating sugar sandwiches when there was nothing else to put between two pieces of white bread.

There were some bright spots, though. For instance, sometimes in the summer we would stay with our Aunt Francis and Cousin Jenni in the country outside of town known as Rose Hill. Jenni owned a small store that was a gathering place for blacks and the core of the Rose Hill community. On Sunday after church, the store was the most crowded, and it was the place we kids grouped together, eating candy and playing.

Aunt Francis was a big woman who could cook anything and always wore an apron. I see her as Aunt Jemima from the syrup ads because she always had a bandanna on her head. We would listen to her ghost stories at night and her tales about working the cotton fields in the daytime. She was always rubbing us down with her healing herbs if we were sick. Aunt Francis had a garden around her house, and most of the food we ate came from her land. I can't remember opening a can of anything. We were shooed away from playing near the vegetable gardens, but we had chores like feeding the chickens and hogs, gathering kindling and wood for the stove, helping churn butter, and making ice cream. When we weren't doing chores, we played tag outside, running and chasing each other. Although we were poor, those times we stayed with Jenni were the most healthy and wholesome of our young lives.

Back at home in town, my mother was always exhausted from childrearing and working the night shift at Goldie's Trail Bar-B-Que. She was 5 feet 2 inches tall and weighed well over

200 pounds. I can't remember a time I saw her happy. She was always yelling at us. Perhaps the lingering memory of being abandoned by her own mother as a child kept her sad, upset, and confused.

In one of her confused moments, I was hurt badly in a kitchen accident. With so many young kids to control, she had a habit of throwing a shoe at us when we were rowdy or disobedient. One time she meant to throw her shoe at me but instead threw the butcher knife in her other hand that she'd been using in the kitchen. I don't remember what happened, but my siblings tell me I was taken to a veterinarian—maybe because there were no doctors close to us, maybe because good doctors didn't treat black folks back then. I don't think I'll ever know for sure. The veterinarian bandaged my wound, but the bleeding would not stop, so they finally took me to the hospital. The emergency room doctor told my family that the knife came 2 inches from my heart.

My mother must have been sick for a long time before she finally went to a doctor herself, but by then the cancer that started in her uterus had spread throughout her body. Her only relief was a morphine drip. They gave us her cancer diagnosis, and she was dead within months. She was only 39 years old.

She died when I was in seventh grade, and that's when I quit school. There was no one to tell me to keep going. My father's presence in our lives was random at best. I still can't tell for sure if there were simply too many of us for him to support or if he just up and left us. I want to believe he could not get help, so he did the best he could by dropping off a couple bags of groceries to the house once a week. It was never enough though, so we quickly learned to steal bread and whatever other food we could lift from the local Piggly Wiggly grocery store as a way to feed ourselves. We were left to raise each other, a pack of children with no guidance.

My sister Pat and I were just becoming teenagers in the

midst of all this, and we were drawn to what we thought was the exciting world of the juke joints, where we could get the attention of adults, mostly men. An older man—he was 21, I was 14—wanted to be my boyfriend, and I was grateful for the attention. He asked me to dance, and I said yes, both of us smiling, me out of shyness.

I had never been told about sex or contraception, and I got pregnant. I knew even less about being a wife and mother, but because I had been to church often as a child, I did believe my boyfriend was supposed to honor God and marry me because I was carrying his child. My upbringing in Rose Hill Baptist Church helped frame my faith. I know for sure that my faith, even though sometimes it has been as small as a mustard seed, has seen me through many storms.

I was 15 when I got married to that man. But he left me soon after, so I was alone with a baby to raise. I moved to California, partly to escape him for good and partly because I heard some cousins in California say that welfare there offered enough money to actually live on. So I packed up my 3-year-old baby girl and got on a Greyhound bus, with just a phone number in my pocketbook. No one knew we were coming.

Eventually my daughter and I landed in the San Francisco Bay Area, where we stayed with some cousins who lived in Richmond. I didn't have much education, but I had always enjoyed learning and reading whatever I could. I enrolled in night school at Richmond High to get my GED. One day at the welfare office I saw a flyer for a job-training program at Linton Business College that was free to welfare recipients. They paid for your childcare and lunch, which is what made it possible for me to enroll. I signed up right there.

My cousins thought I was crazy. "What do you want to do that for?" they said. "If you get a job they'll cut your welfare." But I didn't want to sit on the steps in front of the apartment day after day, bored and singing the blues. More than anything, I didn't want that kind of future for my daughter. So I went to the training program and I never missed a class. I learned everything I could about bookkeeping and typing.

As serious as I was about having a better future, keep in mind that I was 19 and still wanted to get out and kick up my heels, so on the weekends I would go to parties with a girlfriend of mine I'd met while attending Linton Business College. Her name was Cynthia. She was beautiful with short hair, thin like me, but had no children. She had fancy clothes and rode in nice cars—a reality I did not understand, but felt mesmerized by.

I graduated from Linton in June of 1975 and applied for various jobs, but nothing came through. One day I was out of money and my daughter needed something to drink, so I fell back on what I had done to get by growing up. This time I got arrested for shoplifting a carton of milk. Luckily, it was my first time, so I was able to avoid jail by doing some community service. The whole experience scared me so badly that I never shoplifted again.

Eventually I got a job in San Francisco at Bank of America under a federal program to foster equal opportunity for minorities and women. I started at the bank as a clerk typist and later was promoted to trust administrator, investing money for cities and counties. Because I was black and female, employers who wanted to comply with the Equal Employment Opportunity Act that passed in 1972 saw me as a favorable applicant. I think at no other point in history would a single, black mother who had gotten her GED while on welfare have been considered so highly employable. I'm thankful for that opportunity.

Working at a bank, I was around real wealth every day, exposed to people who had estates and second homes and trust funds for their children. I wanted to know what all that was like, and I thought if I had nice things, I would be the kind of person others immediately respected and admired.

Looking back, I understand how naive I was, but you know, we all have to live and learn.

My friend Cynthia quit the college, and I did not see much of her after that. On occasion she would show up at my apartment and ask if she could stay for a while. She never stayed long. Cynthia slept during the day while I went to work.

So, when I first heard Cynthia was found dead on the side of the road—her killer never found—and had been a prostitute, I felt ignorant as I thought about the secret she had kept from me. I never even knew Cynthia's last name. I knew she lived with her sister, liked to listen to Chaka Khan, took black pills, and enjoyed singing. She would argue often with her sister and storm from the house with me trailing after her. Her sister told me once, "Don't get messed up in what Cynthia is doing," but never said what she was doing, and I never dared to ask.

The closest I'd come to being around prostitution was my cousin who danced in a strip club in San Francisco. She never talked much about what she did; she only told me, "It's not for you."

Three years later, when I was 24, I met Sheila. We both worked in San Francisco and had a routine of driving into the city on Fridays and taking the bus on weekdays. Commuting together on Fridays, Sheila would take me to bars in Oakland, introducing me to life in the fast lane. After a few months of driving together, Sheila informed me she was going to quit her job and wouldn't be riding with me anymore. She had met someone.

When I saw her again, maybe 6 months later, she had a new car, lived in a gorgeous high-rise apartment in the Oakland hills, and dressed in nice clothes. It was then that Sheila told me about the world of legal brothels in Nevada.

I knew too well that prostitution was potentially dangerous. But, at the same time, it planted a seed in my mind—here was an opening to possibility, a path to get the kind of money that could change my life forever. My friend's life seemed glamorous, at least from the outside. Illegal prostitution, it seemed, was an avenue taken by women with no skills, whose only other options were to clean rooms in motels, work in restaurants as short order cooks, or just stay on welfare. But this world of legal brothels seemed different.

Even though I had a job and a good apartment outside of Richmond, I was still struggling to pay the rent and cover childcare, medical bills, and transportation into San Francisco. When my car broke down and required hundreds of dollars to fix, it felt to me like I was always one broken-down car away from the life of poverty I had come from. I refused to go back to Mississippi defeated. I didn't ever want to go backward. I wanted to put poverty so far behind me that my daughter and I would never, ever be in danger of slipping back into it.

I already knew that to survive you have to make tough choices and do things you never would imagine doing. Cynthia's death scared me, but didn't stop me. I knew I didn't want to do anything illegal, and I wanted to be as safe as I could be within that dangerous business.

I decided to go to Nevada to work as a prostitute in a legal brothel—a job that paid three times what my bank job did.

It was the summer of 1979. I packed up our things and sent my daughter to stay with my father—who was doing better and living in St. Louis, Missouri—and then I took the bus to Nevada, where I knew the industry was regulated. Under Nevada law, anyone applying to work at a brothel must be checked for sexually transmitted diseases by a doctor and have a criminal history background check, which looks at everything from traffic violations to federal offenses. Once cleared by the state department of health and the sheriff, you are fingerprinted and issued an ID to legally be employed as a working girl—which is the term used in the industry instead of prostitute.

Kitty's Guest Ranch was a new brothel, located just

2 miles outside of Carson City. The house was named after its legendary madam, Kitty Bono. Kitty's had about 20 rooms and a girl in every room. Sofas lined the walls, which were decorated with pictures of partially nude women. The girls wore the trendiest, sexiest fashions, from silk dresses with rhinestone bottoms to hot pants and tank tops. Each girl was required to work 12- to 16-hour shifts nonstop for 3 weeks, and only then take a vacation.

My shift began at eight at night and went until eight the next morning. The first night, I sat dressed and ready, talking with other working girls about how they had entered the business. Behind the beautiful clothes and pretty faces were upsetting stories of abuse, drug and alcohol addiction, and controlling pimps. Their stories made me realize that my story of working at a bank and having my own apartment and car sounded tame.

The night wore on, and no man had chosen me. I was wide-awake at the end of my shift, feeling a lot of doubt about my choices. The rest of the ladies lay sleeping on the sofas, exhausted from their work. Just as I rose to clock out of my shift, the doorbell rang. The hostess yelled "Company, ladies!" giving us time to straighten ourselves up. Suddenly, I became determined to accomplish what in the industry is called "break luck" before my shift ended. I knew I was unskilled compared to the other working girls, and I did not understand the hustle in a lineup. I stood in line with my hands behind my back and said only my name—as I had done all night—but this time I said it with a big smile.

You might find this next part hard to believe, but it's true: The man with the beard who looked like Kenny Rogers, minus the white hair, picked me right away. His name was Jim Fondren. When we were alone together, he told me I was sweet and wonderful. He admitted to me it was his second visit ever to a brothel and he was scared. He fell in love with me after our first visit—I couldn't believe it myself. Who would imagine a man could love you not only after a first visit but also in that context? And yet, he did, as he has proven every day for the past 29 years. He's been a consistent and loving husband, as well as a father figure to my daughter, every step of the way. Jim is the great joy of my life. He calls me a diamond in a sea of sand. I never knew love like this. He saw in me what I did not see in myself.

After learning the business, I left Kitty's so Jim and I could open our own brothel, knowing how lucrative it could be. Jim went through extensive FBI background checks and invested all his money in building the new Sagebrush Ranch. He quickly ran out of money, so we moved from an apartment to a trailer on the construction site.

Jim's mother—a petite blond-haired, blue-eyed woman—came to our trailer to question Jim's new investment. I thought she was beautiful when we met. She wore a hooded coat draped with fur that made her look like a movie star from the '50s. However, she was rude to me and quickly dismissed me from their presence.

After Jim and I married in 1984, he sadly gave up his relationship with his mother to be with me. Our love was colorblind and he tried to get his mother to understand this, but she disowned him anyway.

What I have come to know for sure is to never give up on change. We were not your typical married couple and I felt sorry for Jim; I had learned from my grandmother that you only have one mother, and you cannot replace her. Because Jim is an only child, I sent greeting cards every year to his mother for Christmas, Easter, Mother's Day, and her birthday, sometimes without him knowing.

Several years later, she asked to meet me. Eventually, I was introduced to the rest of her family and friends. We had a loving mother-and-daughter-in-law relationship until the day she died.

While we built the brothel business together, Jim also

went back into real estate development, the work he knew best. In 1984 we had the idea to build a subdivision of homes in a town known for its brothels and gambling. We wanted to offer first-time buyers a chance to own a home and a lot at an affordable price. In addition to the subdivision, we built a number of other businesses: a cable TV company, a Mexican restaurant with a limited gaming license for slot machines, a mobile home park, a sewer treatment plant, commercial and industrial buildings, and several self-storage facilities.

It made sense for me to continue to operate the Sagebrush Ranch, but I brought in a manager to help handle the business. I had worked with prostitutes who were psychologically broken, and I knew for some of them the brothel was their only home. I knew these women wanted to turn their lives around but needed guidance on how to get out and gain more self-confidence.

I held motivational meetings once a week, brought in speakers from the health department, and helped the women file their taxes. I wanted them to go back to school and pick up a trade, buy real estate, open a small business, pursue their dreams. I wanted them to know they would not have to do this forever.

I was trying to help one lady leave her pimp. She was depressed and cried often. One morning, she reached her lowest point and attempted suicide, leaving a note addressed to me that said, "Linda, I'm sorry." Even though she survived, the episode was devastating to me.

There are so many stories and experiences that led me out of the business. It seemed hypocritical to want to help these women by providing a safe place for them to work, yet to use prostitution as a way out of poverty. In 1992 we sold the business. We no longer felt we belonged in that industry, and our real estate business was thriving.

For 20 years we worked hard together, and we were very successful. My daughter's future was secure. We were in a position to sit back and enjoy the benefits of our hard work, and we did just that for a while. We traveled all over the world. I got certified as a captain by the United States Coast Guard to operate a 100-ton vessel, and Jim and I enjoyed exploring the waters of the Caribbean, Canada, and Mexico on our yacht, named Linda Faye. We were rich beyond our wildest dreams. Besides the yacht anchored in the Bahamas, we still own a villa in Mexico and a house in Lake Tahoe, but perhaps I am most proud of owning Magnolia Plantation in Vicksburg, a former working plantation in the slave-owning days. If that isn't a reversal of history and of fortune, I don't know what is.

As wonderful as it was to travel and enjoy our success, on another level I was restless. In the midst of the most luxurious vacations, where the only sound was the sea slapping the sand, I would find myself waking up dreading the day ahead. I found that my days, though full of the kinds of leisure I had always dreamed of, left me feeling empty. I wanted to come back to Vicksburg because I felt that we could make a difference in the town, starting businesses in an area that has been economically depressed for decades. Also, I wanted to be near my family. Today, nine of my family members work with us in the various businesses we opened in Vicksburg.

Do I regret any of my decisions? No. I did the best I could with what I had, given the place and time I was born into. Nothing in my life was ever handed to me. From an early age, I knew that if I wanted my dreams to come true, I was going to have to get busy and work hard to make them happen. These experiences and the choices I made, right or wrong, shaped the person I am today. However, understand that I would not choose the same path for other young women. I have come to know my own power and the power each of us has as our birthright, but I don't want other women to have to travel down the road I did in order to learn that important lesson. I have, as the residents of Vicksburg have come to know, dedicated myself to empowering people.

When I became a top 10 CNN Hero in 2010 along with Anuradha Koirala, who went on to become the Hero of the Year for her crusade to help women in prostitution by raiding brothels in Nepal, it conjured up memories of the Sagebrush Ranch. I wanted to walk up to her and tell her I once owned a brothel and could relate, but instead I told her I had visited Nepal and we only hugged. I told myself I had left that life behind me and it was no longer relevant, so best to leave it in the past.

Then in 2013 I ran for mayor of Vicksburg, and I had to bring my past to light. Although I didn't win, I found people were overwhelmingly positive about my efforts to provide others with the opportunities and choices that did not exist for me. My past, with all its blemishes and complications, helped pave the way for the path I would eventually find with Shape Up Sisters.

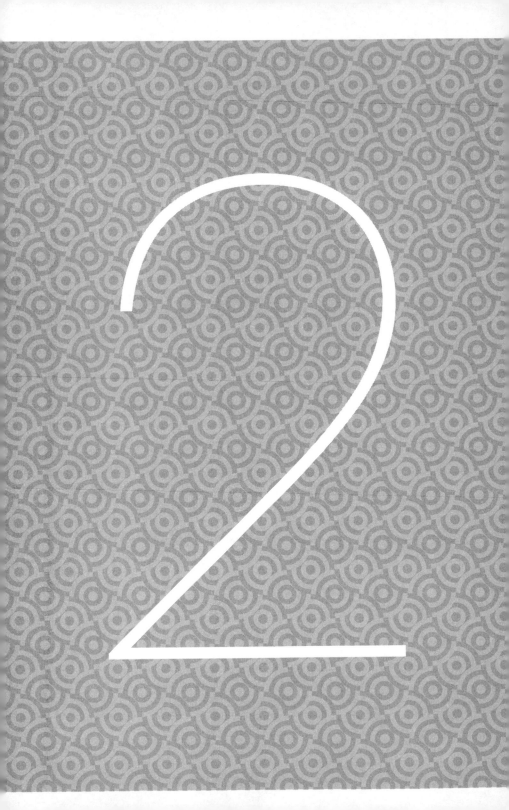

Creating Shape Up Sisters

ALTHOUGH I HAD FOUND LOVE AND FINAN-
cial success in my life, it wasn't until the death of
one of my sisters in 2006 that I discovered my
true passion.

Just before my sister Mary Washington's 54th birthday, I
sat at her bedside as she lay dying. Mary was barely 5 feet tall
but weighed 260 pounds. She was a single mom with two
daughters and three grandchildren. Mary worked constantly,
stringing together various jobs in the food service industry to
make ends meet. She took no time for herself, always working,
cooking, and then collapsing on the couch in exhaustion. I
had tried to encourage her to lose weight by walking with her
in the park, sharing childhood memories together so walking
did not seem like another job. The walks encouraged her, but
when I left to travel, her motivation left too. She refused to go
to a gym and turned down my offer to pay for bariatric surgery. She thought she didn't have time for "all that."

Mary was a cafeteria manager for a school district for 20 years. She loved talking to the children and teachers as they came through her lunch line. She also performed odd jobs on weekends, like fixing hair and catering weddings, funerals, and birthdays. And she worked at events for special needs children every year. When Mary saw a child or elderly person in need, her door was always open and food was always on the table. She did not realize that you could take care of others while also taking care of yourself.

And now it was too late. A brain tumor had ravaged her body, mind, and spirit. I had to lean close to hear her voice. In slurred words she confessed to me, "Linda . . . I wish I had lived my life more for myself."

A sense of sorrow overtook me and I cried for days afterward, thinking again of our mother, who had died at the age of 39, leaving behind 11 of us ranging from ages 3 to 18. Cancer was listed as the cause of death for both my sister and my mom, but in truth, the monster that is obesity was really what had stolen their lives so young.

Fueled by a lack of physical activity and unhealthy eating habits, being obese means more than just carrying around an unhealthy amount of body fat. For Mary and so many of the women I have worked with now, it also means carrying around chronic stress and regret. And it means these women are often sidelined in their own lives. For example, things that people of average weight take for granted were struggles for my sister. Mary never wanted to visit relatives who lived outside of Mississippi because she was embarrassed about not fitting into an airline seat. She didn't like to go to restaurants because she felt self-conscious. It was difficult for her to find clothes that fit.

When Mary confessed on her deathbed, with profound regret, that obesity had robbed her of the ability to live her 54 years to the fullest, I knew I had to do something to help women like her pursue a new path. No woman should have the kind of regret my sister took to her grave.

Although I have lived most of my life at an average weight, that doesn't mean I've never struggled to shed a few extra pounds. In my late 30s, I began to feel flabby; my body was reshaping itself around my belly and hips, and my clothes became a little snug. I had read that life going into middle age isn't smooth. It has bumps and hollows. So I started reading fitness magazines and self-help books, buying exercise videos, and paying attention to any information I could find about healthy eating and exercise.

Following advice from some of the books I read, I set down these goals for myself: exercise three times a week and learn to cook healthy foods. Well, I started and stopped, started and stopped. Each time, I could see a little clearer the barriers associated with my old habits. Finally, by age 40, my efforts led me to a lifelong commitment to my own well-being.

After Mary's death, I realized I had the keys right in my pocket to raise self-awareness and help cure the curse of obesity that cripples so many women in my community. I thought, "What if I could create a social environment in a gym, where exercise does not feel like another form of stress, like I had done with my walks with Mary?"

Six months after Mary's death, I opened Shape Up Sisters and gave it the slogan "Positively Reshaping Women." The aim was to make it an oasis of support and positivity. I instructed the staff to be friendly and welcoming to everybody who came through the door, and to talk to the women throughout their workouts. I knew that heavy women weren't comfortable working out in "hard body" environments (my sister Mary never wanted to go into a gym because she felt people would stare at her). These are women who are not confident when it comes to their bodies. Just fitting into chairs is a struggle for a lot of them. But I believe if there is one health commandment, it is this: *Exercise is the gateway to changing so many things in your life for the better.* Going from being sedentary to being even moderately active delivers immediate benefits, including increased energy, improved mood, and a feeling of mastery over yourself and your surroundings.

Women who came to Shape Up Sisters loved the support and motivation we gave, and they told their friends. I needed to expand my fitness knowledge and make the gym even bigger and more social for these women. Putting my real estate knowledge together with my fitness know-how, I became certified as a personal trainer and purchased a bigger building.

We brought in granite countertops for the reception desk, put in a fruit smoothie bar, got the best equipment available, painted the gym in lovely colors, and didn't scrimp on a luxurious locker room for primping. We also put in a playroom for the kids and offered free childcare.

Talking to the women who came through our doors convinced me more than ever that in the fight against obesity, our main enemy is not body fat itself. It's lack of time, money, and attention that keep people locked in their unhealthy lifestyles. I've hit this wall again and again in Vicksburg. In order to make a change in their lives, women have to believe that change is possible.

From my experiences as a gym owner, I know that it is difficult for women to conceptualize what being healthy looks like. It seems that anywhere you look, the most prevalent examples are either women just like you or the celebrities on television and in magazines. You begin to think overweight women are the norm and women of normal weight are too skinny. Weight loss even becomes a sign of illness. I'll never forget talking to one woman who said she didn't want to start any rumors by losing weight: "I don't want them to say, 'Look, she got AIDS.'"

It's hard to argue with ignorance, but inch by inch we can help people see that they can change their lives for the better. My experiences in Vicksburg have taught me a few things: The underserved community is exactly that: underserved. Lack of time, lack of money, lack of understanding, lack of healthy food sources, lack of self-confidence, lack of good role models—all these things are intertwined and they conspire against us. Most of us are squeezed financially and busy beyond capacity, with spirits so depleted that we have persuaded ourselves we have no time, space, or energy to undertake anything. And when I say this, my intent isn't to discourage you or give you a reason not to follow through. It's just the opposite. People have to know what they're up against.

These women who came to my gym needed a safe, encouraging environment in which to feel confident and create change for themselves. A place where they could be around people who looked like them and faced the same obstacles.

And Shape Up Sisters' programs have proven to be efficient. My employees, whom I call motivators instead of trainers, are all women. Our group fitness classes are packed because we provide women with simple, fun exercises that give them a social experience. There are no barriers: There are no men, so women don't have to feel self-conscious about their appearance or less physically able, and we embrace women of all ages and fitness levels.

Initially I thought we would cater mainly to an African American population. Reports show that overweight and obesity are progressing more quickly among women than men, but that's not all: By 2030, it is estimated that 96.9 percent of African American women will be overweight! And sure enough, black women came. But white women came, too. Hispanic women came. Women of various nationalities came. It was truly a rainbow coalition of women united in their desire to feel better and look better.

Once I had achieved the goal of getting women to be a part of Shape Up Sisters, I realized it wasn't enough. There was more to do. So much more.

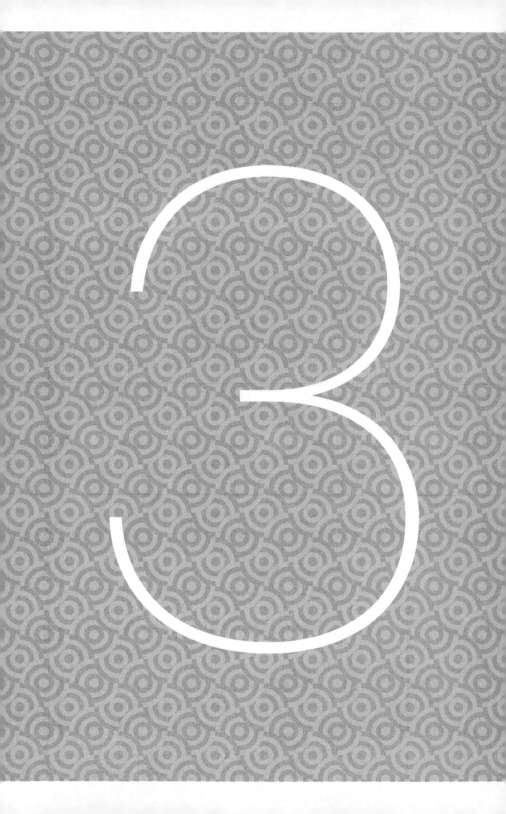

How My Town Lost 15,000 Pounds

L ITTLE DID I KNOW THAT WHAT I WAS INSPIRED to start after Mary's death would not only change a few dedicated gym goers, but would also launch me on a crusade to help the entire city.

I could see the gym offered a new way for women going through the same thing to connect. Suddenly, they were having a shared experience and a conversation. There was a lot of laughing going on, too.

"I lost 200 pounds," I heard one woman say to another.

"Girl, go on!" the other said. "How'd you do that?"

"I left my husband!"

I swear sometimes they exercised more stomach muscles with jokes than they did doing crunches in the aerobics classes. But that was all good. They brought their daughters and their friends and their coworkers and signed them up for memberships. They began making dates to go walking together on the outside track we built next to the gym. And they were so busy laughing and chatting that they didn't even realize they were getting healthy in the process.

One woman I call Mama Coomes—because she treats me like one of her 12 children—serves as an inspiration to other women. At 80 years young, she is now the most popular dancer for the United Way's local version of *Dancing with the Stars*. She is so appreciative of her life and has such a positive attitude. She helps teach the young ladies to stick with exercise and be happy, and she gives out big hugs to the women just for being there that day. Mama is a constant reminder that life at any age is joyful.

All of this started me thinking: It was great that all these women were coming together to help each other tackle mutual issues, but Shape Up Sisters was a little bubble sealed off from the rest of their lives. When they went home, they were returning to the same jobs, the same families, the same couches, the same kitchens, and the same deep fryers—the whole culture that had gotten them fat to begin with.

Remember, this is the South. I think we invented the idea of comfort food. People around here grow up eating fried chicken, fried catfish, fried green tomatoes, mashed potatoes, and biscuits and gravy. From barbecues to buffets on the riverboat casinos, pretty much all of our social functions are tied up with eating and more eating.

Vicksburg has a church on nearly every corner; we are truly the buckle of the Bible Belt. Fellowships and church gatherings aren't limited to Sundays. The pastor's anniversary, revivals, praise dances, Bible studies, family empowerment weekends, special communions, parades, and funerals occur often. Afterward, there's usually a potluck, with these dishes as standard fare: fried chicken, pork ribs, fried catfish, buttered biscuits, mac and cheese, Southern potato salad, corn bread, mustard greens, processed lunchmeat sandwiches on white bread, soda pop, chips, a sheet cake, and—don't forget—sweet tea. Normally I think about what I am putting in my mouth, but when I was running for mayor and going to a lot of these types of gatherings to meet people, I ate the food and shared in good conversations about our community. It gave me a great appreciation for how easy it is to overindulge in fattening food and conversation when you're enjoying fellowship.

At the gym, I started paying attention to the kind of feedback I was getting from the members. They would say things to me like, "I wish my husband would get off the couch!" or "Can my daughter come in and work out with me? She is twice her normal weight."

Then, an article about the health statistics of my state came across my desk. We were number one for the most terrible reasons: Mississippi ranked number one in obesity, number one in poverty, and number one in lack of physical activity. Maybe worst of all, we were number one in infant mortality.

I thought, "This is unacceptable. Enough is enough."

And it hit me: Just like the church potlucks, Shape Up Sisters is its own type of social function—a fellowship, if you will—but one built around exercise and eating healthy. What if it were possible to expand beyond the doors of Shape Up Sisters and create a health-conscious, social environment for everyone in the community? What if everywhere they looked people saw encouragement for healthy living? What if they were given education about healthy choices and had an opportunity to get fit and keep track of their weight? What if I created a fellowship of health and fitness that was free to everyone?

I had heard of a well-known study that looked at whether obesity is contagious. The results of the study indicated that people's weight is very influenced by the appearance, habits, and behaviors of those around them. This means, for example, that if your spouse gains weight, your risk for gaining weight increases. Add to that friends and people you are socially connected to gaining weight, and your risk shoots up astronomically.

What causes this? It doesn't take a genius to figure out that one. You know the old saying, "Birds of a feather flock together"? Well, it doesn't just apply to groups of people; entire regions of the country tend to be similar. High obesity rates are shared in the neighboring states of Alabama, Louisiana, and Arkansas. Just a few years ago, Mississippi was the only state whose obese population topped 30 percent; now there are 13 such states across the country with obesity rates equal to or greater than 30 percent.

It just makes sense that obesity can spread from person to person through social contact. If your friend is overweight and the type who says, "Let's go for hamburgers and a beer after work," you adapt to that. If she has flesh spilling over the top of her pants and her thighs rub together, that can change your idea of what an acceptable weight is. If you gain weight and look like your friend, the extra weight can seem normal to you.

So if that is true, then why can't the opposite be true? If your friends exercise and eat nutritiously, then won't you? I didn't look at any research to see what experts said about that one; it just seemed like that rare thing, common sense. It turns out, however, this has been studied too. In their book *Thinfluence*, authors and Harvard Medical School professors Walter Willett and Malissa Wood note that "social contagion, it turns out, can be a vehicle for positive behaviors as well." The authors go on to say that the decisions we make just for ourselves can "influence those we know, and they can spread even further beyond our social circles, perhaps even beyond our communities, potentially influencing people to whom we may never even be introduced."

Together we can do far more than we can alone, so if together we got moving and ate better, we could lose weight, improve or altogether stop problems like diabetes and high blood pressure, and feel energized. There is a quote by Edward Hale, an American author and historian, that speaks to this: "I cannot do everything, but I can do something. And I will not let what I cannot do interfere with what I can do." Together we could Shape Up Vicksburg!

To make that kind of change, I needed help from some friends, like Bruce Bobbins, a communications specialist in New York who helped me craft a plan. I started to tell people my idea. The most common reaction was, "Why you, Linda?" Why did I choose to tackle the big elephant in the room? My reply was, "Why not me?" Why not anyone? Anyone can start something for others. As a matter of fact, everyone can. If we don't do the things that need to be done and say the things that need to be said, we become part of the problem. Mary's death had made obesity personal to me, and it brought home the depth of the issue. I didn't start a gym to make money, and I wasn't starting this to make money. I wanted to help because it was needed and continues to be needed—desperately. My sister Mary and everyone like her needed this.

Life had taught me that to accomplish anything you need three ingredients:

- Desire
- A motivating purpose
- Faith

For Shape Up Vicksburg, I had all three. It was time to get moving.

It took 3 solid months of passion, planning, and persistence to develop the Shape Up Vicksburg challenge. I knew I wanted to hit three goals:

1. Get people to lose weight
2. Ensure every resident in our city and county became physically active and educated about healthier food choices so that eating right and exercise would become as automatic as putting on a seat belt
3. Make Vicksburg the fittest city in Mississippi

I knew my ultimate goal of claiming the title of Mississippi's fittest city was a long way away, but first things first: How many pounds should the community lose? I didn't want to have folks fixated on an impossible number. Nobody needed to get beaten down by more failure. We all needed success.

So the question was: How should the challenge for time spent and pounds lost be set? Statistics from the Centers for Disease Control and Prevention indicate that two-thirds of adults are overweight or obese. That's two out of every three of us! So I settled on 17,000, a symbolic number representing roughly two-thirds of Vicksburg's population, according to my rough calculations of the Census Bureau's population figures. I also decided that the challenge would be run for 17 weeks, a length of time that was long enough to learn new habits. Seventeen weeks would give the participants enough time to think about what they eat, change how they eat, and increase their physical activity. I did not want this to be a crash diet that lacked proper nutrition. I wanted to start something that would get people to drop weight in a way that they could sustain and manage over time. According to a study in the *European Journal of Social Psychology*, a positive daily action, like eating fruit at lunch or walking for 15 minutes, took an average of 66 days to become as much of a habit as it would ever become. The length of our challenge would be well beyond that.

The established recommendation for weight loss from the National Institutes of Health states that 0.5 to 1 pound per week makes for healthy and sustainable weight loss. I settled on stopping weight gain as a minimum goal, and once that was achieved, I'd aim for each participant to lose just half a pound during the challenge. Research shows that even a 5 to 10 percent drop in weight will improve health, like lowering blood pressure and blood sugar levels that can lead to diabetes. If participants became active and started to watch their diets, they'd probably lose even more. Slow and steady can win the race: Just as we don't tend to notice that creeping weight gain has made us overweight, incremental losses over time add up to significant results.

This weight-loss challenge would need to offer support at every turn. And so along with a team of dedicated volunteers, I created a calendar of exercise events, walks, nutritional and stress workshops, and behavior modification classes. People who signed up could even log on and track their progress at shapeupvicksburg.com.

I knew it was a good plan. But I certainly couldn't mobilize this community effort alone.

First, I had to enlist the support of the City of Vicksburg Board of Mayor and Aldermen. Michael Mayfield, one of our two aldermen, is a 6-foot-tall African American man with an inflated midsection. It seemed that all the food he ate went right to his belly. Alderman Mayfield, who greeted me with a deep Barry White–type voice when I arrived for our meeting, immediately saw the merit of a weight-loss challenge, adding that he wanted to lose 20 pounds of his own toward the total. As we spoke of his love of down-home cooking, he opened a can of Orange Kist soda and poured a packet of salted peanuts into it, a common thing to do around these parts. I knew that if he just replaced that drink with cold water and walked around the block a few times every day, he'd lose those 20 pounds in no time.

I was new to navigating through town politics, and Alderman Mayfield told me that I needed to present the challenge to the city board. If there's one thing I have learned through this process, it's that when you don't know something, ask someone who does.

A few weeks later, I made my case to the board. As I explained the idea of the challenge, many of them started laughing. I didn't get what was funny: Maybe I looked comical dressed up in workout attire with a Shape Up Vicksburg T-shirt rather than typical business clothes. In hindsight, I think it was likely nervous laughter to cover up their discomfort. Apparently nobody had ever stood before them and said they—and their community—needed to lose weight.

"Being the fattest place in America is not the heavyweight title you want to hold," I said. "Citizens look up to elected officials no matter what level the office. When the people see you embark on something positive, they will likely want to follow." I also reminded them that they had taken an oath as elected officials to serve our community.

The city and county board signed on to the weight-loss challenge, as did Vicksburg's then-mayor, Paul Winfield, who—as a young guy and a former high school athlete—also saw the program as a progressive move for the city.

With the elected officials on board, I knew it would also help to win the support of influential members of the community.

Propelled by this exciting momentum, I sought out the CEO of River Region Medical Center, which serves Warren County. I told him I saw little hope in using the challenge to change lives without being able to persuade people to take better care of themselves. I'd grown so used to hearing people ask, "Why go to the trouble of eating well and exercising if you can take a pill to lower your blood pressure and reduce your cholesterol?" Or they'd say things like, "You can count on bypass surgery to save you." We depend so heavily on medications and do not place enough emphasis on preventing diseases through lifestyle changes like eating better and getting active.

We quickly agreed on a partnership in which the medical center would be a weigh-in station and its team of doctors and dietitians would offer free prevention services. Getting information from dietitians about healthy eating was important because our diets are largely associated with diseases such as diabetes, high cholesterol, and hypertension. The hospital would also provide free health screenings so participants could know their numbers for cholesterol, blood pressure, and blood sugar. These numbers would help gauge risk for severe health problems. Truthfully, we should all have an annual checkup, but many of us only make an appointment when we're sick. The challenge was the perfect opportunity to remind people to do that.

Next I met with the manager of Kroger, our biggest local grocery chain, and the general manager of our local Walmart. We discussed how to increase consumers' awareness of what healthy options were already available to them. One idea was to use the "good, better, best" strategy, which helps guide shoppers to healthy, low-calorie choices. For example, whole milk is labeled "good," 2% milk is "better," and skim milk or unsweetened soy milk is "best." The system would work with meat, cereals, and dozens of other foods. I told them that with the help of River Region Medical Center nutritionists, we could also set up walk-throughs with shoppers to show them all the healthy food choices they could make before getting to the checkout counter.

They acknowledged it was worth a try; in addition, the manager of Walmart agreed to set up a free weigh-in station for shoppers.

Now it was on to the schools. I spoke with Gail Kavanaugh,

nutrition director for the Vicksburg Warren School District, who outlined for me all the programs for nutritious eating already implemented in our local schools. "We send material home in students' folders with healthy choices and recipes," she told me. "The problem is that most parents don't bother to look at it."

"All the more reason we need to bring this challenge, and the conversation around it, to the entire community," I replied.

I talked with Ray Neilsen, who, at the time, was chairman of Ameristar Casinos, a large employer in the area, about how offering healthy lifestyle information at work—a small investment in employees' health and fitness—could go straight to the company's bottom line by lowering insurance rates and improving morale and productivity. He wouldn't be the last to see the light. Many local businesses and corporations donated time, money, and products to the challenge.

I also met with church leaders in the African American community because more than half of all the men, women, and children who are overweight or obese are black. After all, if the body is the temple of the Lord, we should treat it with care. They agreed to be a loud voice in this challenge by organizing a gathering of churches to promote physical activity, behavior modification, and access to nutritional foods.

Restaurants—our entertainment hubs around these parts—were another essential part of the campaign. This being the South, where there are more fried-chicken joints and buffet-type restaurants than you can count, we needed to find common ground with the local food establishments. I approached them with a list of suggested menu items, like grilled fish and veggies. A majority of the restaurants already had some items that were in line with the weight-loss challenge, and others changed their menus to offer a few less greasy foods.

Local gyms besides Shape Up Sisters also needed to be involved to help address the overall health of our community. I managed to persuade a few other gyms to allow participants to work out once a week for free and to serve as weigh-in stations during the challenge, which shows how close-knit Vicksburg really is.

Press releases to radio stations, TV stations, and newspapers proved to be a powerful vehicle for getting the word out. The *Vicksburg Post,* our local newspaper, wrote a feature story about the weight-loss challenge; hometown newspapers are good for spreading the word about community events like this because they know the people and the community like no one else. Facebook and the Shape Up Sisters and Shape Up Vicksburg Web sites were great tools for posting messages and updates. Then again, not everyone in our community is computer-savvy or has daily access to a computer. If this event went viral, it was through word of mouth.

I was invited by Christi Kilroy, executive director of the Vicksburg-Warren County Chamber of Commerce, to speak about Shape Up Vicksburg to the local Rotary Club. I emphasized that obesity does not have a color, nor can it choose to be Republican or Democrat. It is multicultural, it is nonpartisan, and it affects us all. The Rotary members were enthusiastic and publicized the challenge in their newsletter.

It was becoming clear to me that good programs and good intentions already existed in our community, but we just weren't implementing them in the most efficient way. The challenge was coming into sharper focus: We needed to coordinate with each other to make the programs that already existed in our schools, businesses, and churches more effective. Shape Up Vicksburg could bring something magical to this community. We could plant something new and thriving—a culture of health and positivity—in the last place people would expect it to grow. And, most important, we could make it happen for ourselves. We had all we needed right in front of us.

An enormous crowd gathered with me for the kickoff event that breezy but sunny autumn morning of October 17, 2009. People of all sizes, creeds, and colors showed up. Men came. Women came, many of them with children. They came with more than just the problem of being overweight: They came with life problems, they came with questions about what they were in for, and, mostly, they came with a willingness to learn how to live a healthier lifestyle.

The morning began with a quarter-mile march from the riverfront murals in downtown Vicksburg to the convention center. We marched to the chant of "Let's shape up Vicksburg." There was live entertainment; free gifts, like water bottles and T-shirts; raffle prizes; cooking demonstrations; Ask-the-Dietitian workshops; health screenings; weight-loss consultations; massages; athletic wear vendors; and, of course, fun outdoor workouts for men, women, and children. It was a unifying experience for the people of our community. It was also the beginning of what I could see becoming a message to carry across the entire state of Mississippi.

U.S. Congressman Bennie Thompson of Mississippi wrote in a letter that I gratefully read to the participants: "It will give families and friends the means of togetherness and exercise." Miss Mississippi of 2009, Anna Tadlock, entertained us, singing the Lee Greenwood song "God Bless the USA." Then-Governor Haley Barbour sent his support for the challenge and Dr. Warren Jones, a family physician and professor emeritus at the University of Mississippi School of Medicine, also stirred up enthusiasm with a chant of "Yes, we can!" State Representative George Flaggs Jr.—who years later would be elected mayor of

Vicksburg—gave a speech pledging $500 to the person who lost the most weight.

You already know that the total weight lost among the participants amounted to 15,000 pounds. Although the average weight loss was 5 pounds, we did not meet our goal of 17,000 pounds in 17 weeks. The timing of our challenge may have been one reason for this. Since most of us gain weight over the holidays, I'd thought that having a start date of October 17 and an end date of February 14 would be ideal for helping us all navigate the season's indulgences, but I was mistaken. The holiday season is such a special time of year, and all that exercise and eating right were drowned out by shopping, celebrating, entertaining, football (and snacking!), old bad habits, and cold weather. The free seminars and exercise events scheduled at community centers, churches, and businesses throughout the 17 weeks were supposed to make it easier for us to come together, but because of all the hustle and bustle of the holidays, they were not as well attended as I would have liked. I racked my brain, asking myself what I could have done differently.

Still, there was so much to celebrate. We gathered together again on a cold, rainy March day to celebrate the ending of the 17-week weight-loss challenge. There was a feel-good fashion show that allowed participants to parade their happiness and model their weight-loss success. There were many feel-good stories of weight loss to applaud that day. There was the 18-year-old mother of two and two-time cancer survivor who had dropped from 230 to 210 pounds (the Mississippi Make-A-Wish Foundation had contacted me to help grant her wish of losing weight). There was a soul food restaurant owner who had lost 30 pounds after he stopped eating his own hush puppies and fried chicken and started walking. What's more, our efforts seemed contagious: I heard about churches that went on "spiritual weight-loss journeys" to shed 1,000 pounds by Easter after hearing about Shape Up Vicksburg, and there was a bank manager who had challenged her tellers to lose weight with weekly meetings after work. My team and I continued to attend health fairs throughout the community and gave talks to Walmart and Kroger employees. There was a woman in my gym that confessed to me that Shape Up Sisters and Shape Up Vicksburg had saved her life. She had been suicidal and an alcoholic for years and had recently quit drinking and smoking. She'd already lost 30 pounds and was now committed to her new healthier life. These are just some of many stories that I heard in the wake of our weight-loss challenge.

But for all of our success, I didn't feel like I had reached enough people. Some confessed they'd thought about joining and hadn't, and some said they hadn't even heard about it, despite all of our promotion.

So I decided to introduce an ongoing Shape Up Vicksburg Get Healthy Walking Club at our local park. The spring months were coming and the weather would be perfect for walking. At our first gathering, I told the crowd that there is no better or simpler exercise for body, mind, and spirit than walking. It's what our bodies were designed to do, and (virtually) anyone can do it

Our motto—"Walking Is Cheap, Life Is Priceless"—was printed on shirts that were given out to anyone who joined us. It worked. One time, a member of my gym was walking through Walmart wearing the T-shirt, and a man approached her and said, "You are right ma'am, life is priceless. My wife has cancer." It brought tears to my eyes when she told me that story. The T-shirts were a reminder to stay persistent. I wanted the men, women, and children of our community to understand that while the weight-loss challenge had officially ended, Shape Up Vicksburg had not. What we embarked on with the challenge was for the long haul, and we were still here to help.

My husband, daughter, siblings, cousins, and their families all pitched in to organize our many activities, working alongside me and adding their energy and dedication to the cause. Where would I be without my family? Let me tell you, I do not take any of them for granted.

We remained determined to continue to increase participation. I kept working on the elected officials and the chief of police to attend our walks, which sometimes attracted upward of 200 people.

When CNN contacted me and named me a Hero, I acknowledged that 15,000 pounds was short of our original goal. But as I said, it was never about the number. Heck, those 15,000 pounds wouldn't have been lost otherwise. More significant was the fact that the community was now working together and creating change. Something had taken root. Skepticism had turned to enthusiasm. Citizens were keeping each other motivated; those in the community who were not overweight encouraged overweight family members and coworkers to get active and eat healthy. Many participants formed smaller groups to motivate and support one another. If that's not an example of a community-wide movement, I don't know what is.

Today, Shape Up Vicksburg continues to draw people to nutrition seminars and organized walks. Best of all, fitness has been woven into the fabric of our community culture.

Getting this challenge off the ground started a conversation not only about how good it feels to be in shape, but also about what makes people fat to begin with and what keeps them fat. Shape Up Sisters is about getting people off of their butts and into the habit of moving, and it's about helping them use food as nutritious fuel, not as comfort or refuge. It's also about respecting life and embracing a positive mind-set.

Even though I'm a gym owner, no gym membership is necessary to achieve any of this. In fact, what I want you to do is to incorporate more movement into your regular life. I want you to learn about how nutritious foods that you prepare at home can help you take back the kitchen and give you and your family greater energy, better health, and stronger, fitter bodies. I'm going to be talking a lot about how to make that happen in the following pages. It starts in your head and goes to your heart. Your head and your heart will work together to get you going—and keep you going.

If you're ready to Shape Up, read on.

Part 2
"Mother Wit": Shape Up Sisters in Action

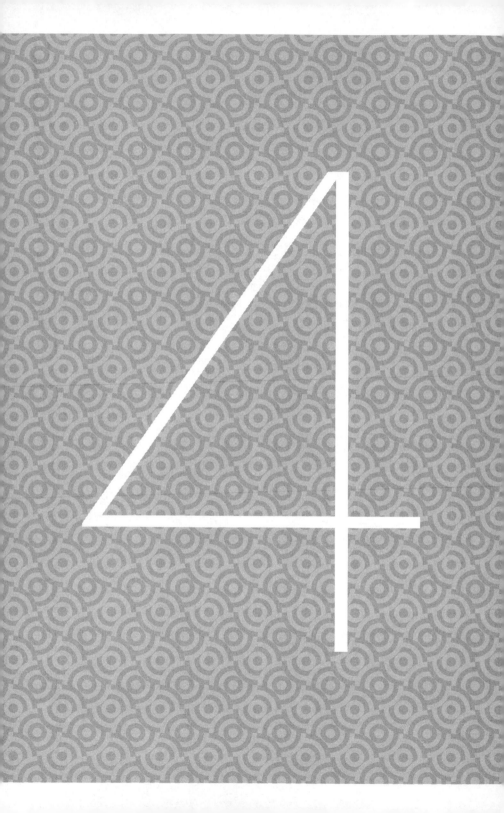

Mother Wit

Awakening the Common Sense
You Already Have

"MOTHER WIT" IS WISDOM THAT COMES from life's journey. It's an expression we use in the black community here in the South, and it is really just another phrase for common sense. This section of the book is about awakening your own Mother Wit—not relying on someone else's account of how you should look and feel and using the right tools to figure things out for yourself.

"She don't have the common sense God gave her" or "Honey, he don't have sense enough to come in out of the rain." How many times have you heard people say something like that? Where I grew up, people put a lot of value not just on book learning, but also on common sense.

Over the years I have gained greater insight into Mother Wit. It has a lot to do with the universal law of cause and effect. Every act of mine—everything I do, say, or think and every emotion I betray—has an impact on those around me.

How do you get Mother Wit? You already have it. You were born with it, and you develop it as you go through life. If you don't feel it now, yours is just hidden or asleep! In the following pages, I will take you on a journey to discover and grow your Mother Wit. You possess value and you need to embrace your power to nurture not only other people but also yourself.

When the late film critic Gene Siskel asked Oprah, "What do you know for sure?" she said the question threw her off. Since then, she has used the question as a way to take stock of her life, and she even created a monthly column in the back of *O, the Oprah Magazine*, titled "What I Know for Sure," to help answer it. I think of her column as a call to awakening Mother Wit. The advice she gives often provokes women to self-reflect and stay true to their values. I always read this column first before continuing with the rest of the magazine. In fact, I was so inspired by the concept of "what I know for sure" that it was the theme of my 50th birthday party.

My own Mother Wit comes from the instincts sharpened in me at a young age by my grandmother. Mama Liza was one of the wisest and oldest of our family members. She held Rose Hill Baptist Church and the family together. She took me in when my mother threw the butcher knife at me and then again when I was too pregnant to care for myself.

She was superstitious; if she found a penny lying heads up, she would put it in her shoe for luck. (I still do this today, a habit I picked up from her all those years ago!) She'd say, "If your left eye is twitching, it means trouble. Beware." We covered the mirrors when there was lightning so as not to attract it. These old ways might not have made much sense at the time, but looking back I can see it was always rooted in something practical—if only to lift our spirits and be attuned to potential danger.

Mama Liza was a small-framed woman who would sleep during the day and do her household chores—while singing—after midnight when it was quiet and the Mississippi summer heat was not so intense. I would lie awake and watch her rub Noxzema cold cream onto her face, then move on to the cleaning, ironing, and sewing.

She had hopes for me—until I got pregnant. Even so, she never shouted at me. She was even-tempered. She used old-time expressions, wise words that have stuck in my head all these years. She would often repeat sayings like, "Get that speck out of your own eye before you try and get it out of anybody else's," "A stitch in time saves nine," "A closed mouth don't get fed." Most of all, she taught me, "Self-preservation is the first law of nature."

"You might not have an education, but you got Mother Wit. You'll be alright," she would tell me assuredly, with a nod of her head.

And you will be all right, too. Go on, now. Turn the page.

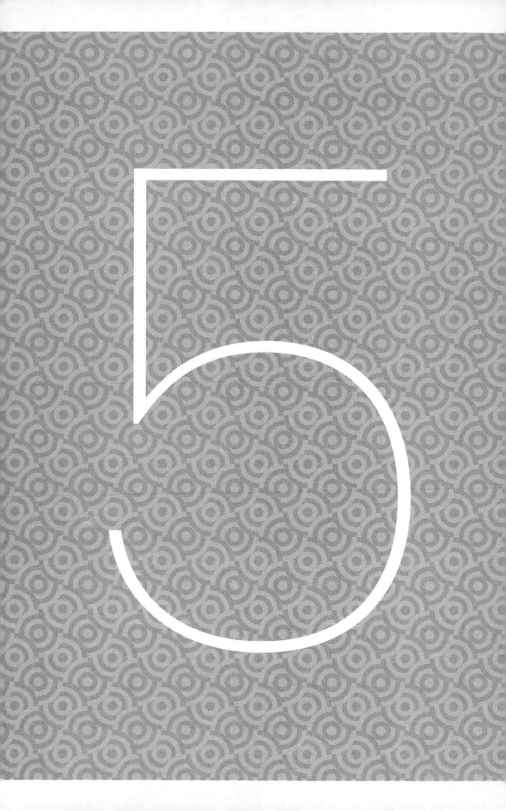

Get That Speck Out of Your Own Eye

Seeing Clearly What Needs to Be Done

YOU HAVE TO LOOK THE FACTS IN THE FACE before you can do anything about them. One of the hardest things to do is critique ourselves. When Mama Liza used to say, "Child, you need to get that speck out of your own eye before you try to get it out of anyone else's," what she meant was that you have to see your own situation clearly.

How clear are you about your health? Do you talk about your health like everything's fine, but know that you could be doing more to feel fit and energetic? Do you shake your head at others for overindulging or being sedentary, but fall back on excuses for not doing more yourself? Do you know you need to lose weight but are afraid that you'll fail again—so you don't try?

Not seeing clearly can lead to inaction, inactivity, and resentment.

Good health will follow when you remove that speck from your eye by tending to your own attitude and assessing what type of change you need to make.

Making the Change

This is a conversation I have had many times with women in Vicksburg:

"How can I stay motivated to lose weight?" they ask.
"By understanding why you gained weight," I say.
"How can I understand it?"
"By not fearing it."
"How do I not fear it?"
"Through action. The best way to conquer fear is through action."

Being honest about what you've been up to is the first step to knowing what actions you need to take next to overcome your situation. These are questions I ask first-time members wishing to join my gym:

- Do you exercise now?
- When was the last time you worked out?
- What type of exercises did you do?
- Why did you stop?

Let me tell you, if our commitment to exercise was as persistent as our excuses, we would all be triathletes. The answers I hear to those questions range from "I used to, but I got bored" to "I don't have a babysitter" to "I lost my job." By far, the most prevalent excuse is "I don't have time." But if you don't make time to exercise, then you'd better schedule in time to be sick.

I know a lady named Michelle. She confided in me about something that has been bringing her down—her home. When she is in someone else's home, she is comfortable because she doesn't feel the need to do anything. But in her own home, she cannot relax because her mind constantly flashes to all the things she *should* be doing: picking up after the kids, cleaning out the closets, straightening the living room, hanging pictures, or doing other chores. I can't do this because I need to do that! But here's the problem: Her mind is so overwhelmed that she does *nothing*. She watches TV standing up because she feels she needs to be doing something, but how useful is that? Not very.

Michelle knows how important exercise is and that it will give her more energy. Yet she can't do it because the confusion in her mind is as big as a mountain—an obstacle blocking everything else. With all of her concerns and worries, not only does Michelle not exercise, but she also doesn't do the other things she *needs* to do because she cannot focus enough to set priorities.

This way of thinking also pervades other areas of her life. For example, she admitted to me that she doesn't date because she feels she should be doing other things, including taking care of her daughter's needs. Small things make Michelle angry and she is constantly irritable.

In response to Michelle's situation, I asked her to take out a piece of paper and write the answers to the following questions and then read them back to herself:

- Are you afraid to ask for help?
- Do you ever sit down to gather your thoughts?
- What are you telling yourself that keeps you from doing what you need to do?

At first she hesitated. "I don't want to write this stuff

down! I don't want somebody to see it and then be all up in my business!"

I told her if she was concerned to just tear it up and throw it away as soon as she was done. Keeping it isn't the point. What matters is the act of writing itself, seeing your thoughts in front of you and being honest about them. Only by getting out what's inside can we start to gain perspective. This is how change can start to take place. You have to create the conditions for change to happen!

Believing the Change

As I told Michelle, after you answer those questions, answer these too:

- What would being healthy look like? How would I dress? What would people say to me?
- What would my day look like if I were doing things to get in better shape?
- What can I change today that will start me on the path to doing that?

The only way positive change can come into your life is if you seek it out, make it a priority, and embrace it. How do you make it a priority? You must first schedule it in like you do with anything else in your life that's important. In the coming chapters you will find many strategies for making this happen, but know this: Exercising and eating nutritious foods are not treats you give to yourself once in a while, nor are they penance for eating that second piece of pie. They are a necessary part of living a full, healthy life. The conversation you have with yourself should change from "If I have time I will exercise" to "I will create the time to exercise" and from "If I have time I will prepare healthy meals" to "I will create healthy meals."

You don't have to solve everything at once. Don't think about the clock. Don't even think about everything you must do: Just do one thing after another. All you need to do is the task right in front of you right now. If you think about life as a series of *I have to get lunch at 1:00, go to a meeting at 3:00, then pick up the kids at 3:30,* you are locked into the clock like a hamster on one of those wheels. Just do what needs to be done and stop giving yourself an extra task to complete; you'll do a better job with everything you do.

Sometimes we get so wrapped up in the illusion of not having time that we waste even more time. If you practice letting go of the clock and just doing what is at hand at this very moment, a magical thing starts to happen: You will actually find more time and feel less confusion. You should not be controlled by thoughts like *I can't exercise because I have to pick up the kids/have a meeting/cook dinner.* Focus instead on the idea that happiness comes from being healthy enough to keep up with those kids, participating actively in the meeting, and enjoying that dinner.

The main reason you do not make fitness and healthy eating a priority is because you are putting energy into too many other things that do not benefit you long-term. Ask yourself if what you are watching on TV is worth 10 years off your life or if talking to that friend who only ever complains about other people is worth the 20 minutes that is sucked out of your day. Let's take that same energy and channel it into self-motivation. Your current health is not due to lack of time or money. It is the result of a series of choices you have made year after year. Now, you might not have known you even had choices, or you might not have realized what you were doing. The goal is to grow past where you are right now. First, you must know where you are! Then, after you know, let it go and move forward.

Tracking the Change

Does your body weight indicate you are above the range for good health? There are several methods out there to determine this. However, I'm not going to talk in a scientific foreign language about how to track all that. Body fat and weight are not the only measures of good health. It is possible to be healthy by *other standards*—cardiovascular fitness and strength—while exceeding the norm for an ideal weight.

I wish you could see through the eyes of women at my gym when they hear their body composition results—known as Body Mass Index—indicate that they fall into the obese category. Many of them have never heard of BMI. They become consumed with sadness and disappointment at this new information. I let them know I am glad they are showing up and that this is only one tool to help them see more clearly what needs to be done.

Still, it's important to have *some* means to track your progress, week after week, so you have feedback for your effort. The simplest way to track your body weight on your own is the tried and true bathroom scale. Don't get too hung up on small gains and losses, as weight can fluctuate from day to day, but schedule a weekly weigh in to be sure you're heading in the right direction.

Now let me introduce a quick and reliable method for determining your body fat distribution. It is called *waist circumference*. The size of your waist is a reliable visual indicator of abdominal obesity. If you gain weight in the abdominal area and develop an apple-shaped body, you are at increased risk for developing heart disease, stroke, hypertension, and type 2 diabetes, certain types of cancer, gout, sleep apnea, and osteoarthritis. Waist circumferences of greater than 35 inches are considered a strong indicator of abdominal obesity in women.

It is meaningful to note that losing just 5 to 7 percent of your body weight can cut your risk of diabetes by nearly 60 percent.

You may ask, "Well, what do *you* know?" One thing I do know from my mother's and sister's experiences and the experiences of many friends and Shape Up Sisters members is this: Being obese is not just a matter of numbers on a scale; it has physical, emotional, social, medical, and psychological effects. You are entitled to more than that. You are entitled to a life in which you can move like you want to move and feel like you want to feel—and nothing less. It is hard work, but we are going to help get you there.

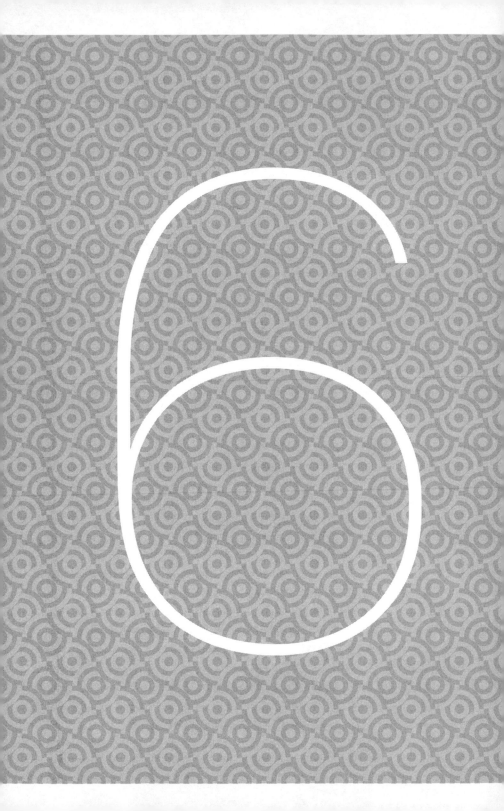

Nothing Beats a Failure but a Try

**Eliminating Obstacles—
and the Basics of Getting Healthy**

"I WILL TRY TO BE CONSCIOUS OF WHEN AND why I eat and will, to the best of my ability, eat simply to satisfy my nutritional needs as opposed to my emotional needs. I will also do my best to make healthful food choices."

These are lines from the Shape Up Vicksburg contract that all our participants signed before starting the challenge. The most important words in the contract are "I will do my best." When you do your best but do not reach your goal, it is not a failure. It is just another opportunity to do better. The next most important words are "be conscious." Being unaware of what and why we are eating, why we avoid exercise, and why we keep doing the same old things is one of the major reasons why we fail. Tuning in to these cues and being truthful with ourselves about these urges and obstacles can help us succeed at finding our way back to better health.

Maybe this sounds familiar to you: You start exercising and eating well, and you're thinking everything will suddenly change. And for a while, it does. You get on the scale and you've lost 5 pounds! But then the days wear on, and it gets harder to follow that diet and to get up and exercise. Before you know it, your motivation has evaporated.

Most women who join Shape Up Sisters say lack of motivation is the number one reason they gave up trying to exercise on their own and walked through the door. But even in the gym, after 2 or 3 months, motivation can start to lag. I start noticing that some women miss a class here or skip a walk there.

I'm not saying issues don't arise in our lives that throw us off track. But when I see a pattern, it usually means something is going on. One thing I've noticed is that as soon as women start making a little bit of progress and start feeling a little bit better about themselves, but maybe also a little bit bored or impatient, those familiar excuses—"not enough time" or "I got hurt"—start popping up like dandelions in spring. (If only they would change up their routine often enough, they would stick with it! But more on that later.)

Another self-defeating pattern I see is women who throw themselves into an exercise resolution and overdo it. There's one woman I know like this—I'll call her Shirley—who just breaks my heart. Shirley is beautiful, with black hair that winds down her back. She works in an office and her job demands a lot of sitting. Shirley sometimes walks with a limp when her knee is acting up. Every pound of body weight puts 5 pounds of force on her knee, so even 10 extra pounds puts a considerable load on her joints. Like so many of us, Shirley has been struggling with her weight—losing it, then gaining it right back. Shirley told me she feared being obese because her family has a history of heart problems, type 2 diabetes, and high blood pressure. She already has two of these diseases. Since no one around her seemed to care about their weight, it was hard to stay motivated to lose the weight that might control her blood pressure and diabetes.

After hearing about Shape Up Vicksburg, Shirley thought maybe it was the motivation she needed to get going. She decided she would aim to lose 50 pounds. She went from eating fried chicken and sitting at home in the evenings to following a 1,000-calorie-a-day diet and working out 7 days a week.

Sure enough, she started to lose weight that first week. Then reality set in.

We spoke on many occasions about her progress. "It's hard to keep going and not break down and quit," she would tell me.

I would suggest to her that she was making it harder on herself than it needed to be, trying to go from 0 to 60 overnight. She had set up an unrealistic diet and a demanding exercise routine that would be hard to maintain over time, given where she was starting. "Create a solid foundation that you can build from," I advised. "You want your weight loss to be successful and permanent. Any dietary strategy and exercise routine can work, if you can stick with it for a lifetime. Don't rush it."

The Centers for Disease Control and Prevention numbers show that only about 5 measly percent of folks who lose weight with a crash diet keep that weight off for any significant amount of time. But she didn't want to hear that. She had been sucked into the "no pain, no gain" attitude that she had seen in countless movies and infomercials. Her idea of good health meant suffering.

She lost 17 pounds by the time the challenge ended, but, sadly, gained it back in short order. Whenever I see her now, she always makes sure to tell me why she is no longer walking and why she is no longer paying attention to what she eats. It's her thyroid, see. It's a bad knee, see. It's just so much stress at work, see. It's that she has a friend coming in from out of town.

I nod and give her a hug. I know that she has within her the ability to change and reach her goal of losing 50 pounds. Each failure teaches you what to do differently next time, until you succeed. But to get there, Shirley will need to be more conscious about what is holding her back and why it is always easier to make an excuse than to commit to change.

Of course I am all too aware that many of the "excuses" we make are not empty excuses, but factors of hard and busy lives. I remember when, in the days leading up to the Shape Up Vicksburg challenge, a group of us visited area neighborhoods to drum up interest. People perched on their porches while kids played in their yards and conversations among neighbors carried on in the driveways. In many ways, the scene seemed like an ideal suburban, apple-pie-in-the-sky setting, but listening in on their conversations, it was clear that money, kids, jobs, and relationships were foremost on their minds. And even though most of the women I met were overweight, "eating right" and "getting fit" were just items at the bottom of a long to-do list. I suspect this is the same with other women across America. Also, it's normal to have negative feelings come up when you're confronted with breaking long and strong habits, like smoking, eating late at night, skipping exercise, overindulging in alcohol, and giving up too easily. Some of the people we spoke with just ignored us or said, "It's none of your business!" But we did find women that day who were inspired by the Shape Up Vicksburg idea. And despite all their fear and their skepticism that something could be different in their lives, they were willing to try.

What I know for sure is that people want to do better, but they need help. We all have many reasons—good and bad—why we aren't doing the things that would make our lives happier, healthier, and more productive. The problem with most diet and exercise advice is that it doesn't acknowledge the real-life barriers that stand in the way of healthy living. It's time we stop pretending and start coming up with solutions that meet folks where they really live so we can break the cycle.

What We're Up Against

I've got to tell it like it is: By most estimates, two-thirds of any weight lost is gained back within 1 year, and almost all of it within 5 years. Why is that? Well, it turns out there are a lot of hidden enemies to fight in the battle of the bulge.

First off, what you inherit plays a big role: In fact, a recent study from UCLA indicated that the degree to which you gain weight is at least in part due to your genes. Granted, the study was done on mice, but it showed that when fed the exact same high-fat, high-calorie diet, some of the mice didn't gain weight, while others saw their body fat increase by 600 percent! Other studies have shown that some people have more fat cells than others, which means they have a natural tendency to hold on to extra fat. For women—who on average have a higher percentage of body fat than men—the situation is even more challenging.

Now don't go thinking there's no hope and that you were just "born this way." Your genes are not your destiny. You might not have been born to be skinny, but everybody can be healthy. Even if you did inherit more fat cells, moving your body changes all that. It's never going to make your fat genes go away, but it will keep them from taking over.

That's where a healthy environment comes in. Weight isn't all determined by genes, but our own biology is programmed to crave energy in the form of sweet and high-fat foods, which used to be very scarce but, in today's food environment, are available everywhere you turn. That's why you can't just rely on willpower to lose weight. If it were that simple, obesity would not now be the number one leading cause of preventable death, even beating out smoking. And for most of us, our willpower also falls prey to negative thinking—worry, fear, loneliness, guilt, anger, resentment, and shame tend to overwhelm our good intentions.

That's why it's so important to put yourself in a more positive environment—surrounding yourself with people who support your interest in better health, avoiding temptation by not bringing home unhealthy foods, and not holding yourself up to unrealistic media images. One of the biggest challenges we face is learning what healthy looks like. Without recognizing what to aim for, it's hard for us to get there, and it's even harder when we are influenced by the media to chase false and unrealistic ideals of beauty.

I can tell you from the experiences of women I've worked with that holding yourself up to an image that just isn't you or aiming for an unrealistic ideal will only hold you back. Sure, Rihanna, Jennifer Lopez, and Jennifer Aniston are all beautiful. But they have access to unlimited resources to help them achieve that glamorous look, as well as an army of people helping them. Remember: You can't be anyone else, and they can't be you. You are unique and beautiful, inside and out. And anyway, when we compare ourselves to an unrealistic ideal like a celebrity, there may be a tendency to think, "I'll never look like that," and instead keep gaining weight with our friends. That's not right, either.

Instead of using celebrities as role models, take some inspiration from real women, like Vicksburg's Evelyn Weaver. She was not obese, but she had struggled with extra weight for over 20 years, since her second child was born. Evelyn tried everything—all the different diets she saw that looked so amazing in commercials—but she was always disappointed with her results. She tried to eat right and always exercised, but the outcome was the same—weight off for a little while and then back on. After having surgery for a medical condition, she shot up to 160 pounds, and the extra weight refused to come off. She was very down on herself. She had no self-confidence and never thought she was pretty or sexy enough. It got to the point where she wouldn't go out because she was sure people were staring at her and snickering, "Look at her." At restaurants she tried to eat small amounts so people would not think she was, as she said, "a pig." She was deeply unhappy with herself.

Evelyn joined Shape Up Sisters, and after several weeks in the gym doing our circuit workout and attending our fitness classes, she lost 15 pounds. She wanted an even bigger challenge and found the courage to join several of our Better Body Bootcamps. Perfect strangers were complimenting her appearance and saying, "I can tell you work out!" She wanted to participate in Shape Up Vicksburg as walking proof of what sticking with a program can do. She is now 137 pounds and a size 8, instead of a size 12. Most of all, she feels good about herself, and her crippling lack of self-confidence is gone—and that is the healthiest thing of all.

Or consider Tonya Perkins' story. Tonya was diagnosed with breast cancer when she was 27. Luckily, 5 years of medication and treatments saved her life. But she went into a funk emotionally, neglecting herself. When she realized her blood pressure was creeping up and her health might again be at risk, she was willing to take the reins. Her doctor told her that buying tennis shoes was the best way to avoid another cancer diagnosis. Tonya joined Shape Up Sisters and has been a regular in our group fitness classes ever since. In the kitchen, she has learned that making easy substitutions to her usual meals—like whole wheat pasta instead of regular spaghetti, and ground turkey instead of beef—can save a lot of calories and boost nutrition.

Evelyn and Tonya were able to get—and stay—healthy by adding more movement to their lives and making simple adjustments to their diets. Unlike our friend Shirley, who went to extremes, these women made their changes in a manageable and consistent way.

Little Changes, Big Results

Trust me, because I've seen it: Little changes do add up. Small and gradual losses, like 10 percent of your weight, give you amazing health benefits—like preventing diabetes, lowering blood pressure, and reducing bad cholesterol—that can be continued over time. And you know what else? You have all you need right now to get to that 10 percent loss—and beyond, if you want to.

You just have to be patient. The experience of Linnie Wheeless, the public relations director of Shape Up Sisters, is a perfect example. This is what she told me:

"When I was in high school, I was 30 pounds heavier than I am now at age 40. I was an athlete and lettered in two sports. People would probably have referred to me as being big boned or having an athletic build, but the truth was that I was overweight. My family ate out every single night. My mom gave up on cooking when I was 13, so for 5 years, every meal except breakfast was at a restaurant.

"I was not happy with my body. Even though I was in very good shape, I did not like to shop for clothes. I wore a much bigger size than my friends. I was an honors student and considered to be quite bright, but I did not understand healthy eating and nutrition. I thought that a sensible diet meant skipping dessert, so I ate barbecue, hamburgers, and pizza and then said no to cheesecake, thinking I would lose weight.

"I remember going to dinner with my dad on one occasion. I told him I was on a diet. When the waitress brought my order of chicken-fried steak and set the plate in front of me, he said, 'That's a diet?' My head dropped in shame. I informed him that I was not getting dessert, but I realized then that what I thought was eating healthy was wrong.

"My freshman year in college was an eye-opening period in my life. When I got on the scale in front of my tennis coach, I broke down in tears. She told me that she could help me with my weight. I was so grateful.

"She gave me a very simple list of goals: Do at least 30 minutes of cardio activity, like walking or dancing, three times a week; do some form of weight lifting two times a week; and eat six mini meals throughout the day rather than three big meals (and never late at night).

"That was it. I followed those rules and my life changed. I didn't avoid foods and I didn't suffer. I started losing weight, about 1 to 1.5 pounds a week. I had more energy and felt better about myself. I naturally became more interested in eating healthy food, and it wasn't hard. In 6 months I lost 30 pounds.

"Twenty years later, I still follow her advice. I've had periods where I gained a few pounds and lost a few pounds, but for the most part, I've stayed fit. I made a lifestyle change when I was young and I have benefited tremendously from that decision."

As you can see from Linnie's story, improving our diets doesn't have to be some difficult, revolutionary change. The trick to eating healthy, nonfattening food isn't a trick at all. Too many diet books offer advice that is simply not realistic for most people, particularly those on a budget. Part 3 of this book contains a more extensive eating plan, but know this: Cutting back on calories and increasing the good stuff—the nutrients our bodies need—boils down to:

- Decreasing the added sugar we take in, especially from sugary drinks like soda pop
- Eating more whole grains, vegetables, and lean meats

That's it. (And yes, I know that fresh produce can cost a lot, but research has shown that frozen and canned produce can be just as nutritious and it costs much less. See page 124 to find out more.)

I'll say it again: One of the biggest challenges we have is learning what healthy looks like. Over the years at the gym, and then through our community challenge, I have heard so many women express confusion about what goals they can realistically set and how to get there. Here are the most common questions I'm asked and my responses. Hopefully they will help you see a way forward.

Getting Healthy 411

Q: How often should I exercise?

A: Physical activity is a matter of life and death. Start by doing what you can and then look for ways to add more. If you have not been active for a while, start out slowly. The Centers for Disease Control and Prevention recommends that you do both aerobic and strength training exercises to stay healthy. For aerobic activity (aerobic simply means "with oxygen"), that translates to, at minimum, 2.5 hours a week of walking, running, biking, or stair climbing. Walking is one of the best ways to add physical activity to your life if you have not been active. It burns 200 calories an hour (more if you haven't been active) and it's what our bodies are designed to do. For the first couple of weeks, walk for 10 minutes a day for 3 days. Then, add more time and days: Try 15 minutes instead of 10, and eventually start walking 5 days a week. Pick up the pace once this is easy for a couple of weeks. You may want to add more activities on weekends for variety.

Once you have been consistent with an aerobic routine,

you are ready for the new challenge of adding weight resistance or strength training exercises two times a week. Weight resistance increases muscle mass, and when you have more muscle, your body burns more calories. It also helps strengthen your bones so you don't develop "brittle bones," otherwise known as osteoporosis.

Q: Is one type of exercise better than another?

A: Do anything you enjoy as long as it gets your heart rate up for at least 10 minutes. Aerobic exercise, also known as cardiovascular exercise, increases your breathing and heart rate, strengthening the heart and lungs. Aerobic exercises include walking briskly, dancing, and running, to name a few.

Keep in mind that all aerobic exercises are not the same: Walking allows you to use your own weight as resistance, so you burn more calories walking than riding a stationary bike, where your weight is supported. This is not to say that riding a stationary bike is not a decent type of aerobic exercise. In fact, it is great for beginners. And if you have knee issues, you may need to support all of your weight by sitting when you first start exercising. But your ultimate goal should be to support your own weight.

Eventually, for a well-rounded routine, you'll want to add exercises for flexibility and balance, too.

Strengthening activities include pushups, situps, lifting weights, heavy gardening (digging and shoveling), or working with resistance bands. If you do aerobic activity without strength exercises, you will burn calories and improve heart health, sure, but you won't be getting stronger, which— believe it or not—affects everything from your posture to your ability to do everyday chores like lifting groceries. (And muscles burn more calories than fat does, even when you're sitting on the couch!) If you choose not to be sedentary and add exercise, you can shave 10 to 15 years off your biological age. It's not just more years; it's more years you can live well.

Q: How long will it take to start losing weight?

A: One to 2 pounds a week is realistic. If you burn 500 more calories than you eat every day for a week, you should lose that much.

Remember to be patient, especially if you have more than 20 pounds to lose. You can't expect a new you in a week. How do you stay motivated to keep pressing on since weight loss is so gradual? In my gym, I hung up a motivational quote defining the word *challenge:* "Undertake something difficult; it will do you good." I urge my members to look at the quotes often—I've got a dozen of them hung on the walls throughout the building. One saying that I find to be absolutely true is "Motivation is what gets you started. Habit is what keeps you going."

They say it takes 21 days to start a habit. If you can try to make exercise as routine as brushing your teeth and as fun as gossiping with a friend (which you can do while you walk), then you will stick to it and you need not worry that the weight will come back. Then, to really make a commitment to your health and hit your goals, see if you can keep it going for 90 days (and sign our Shape Up contract on page 73).

Q: Do I need to join a gym?

A: Think of exercise as an investment: Exercise will improve your productivity at work and it will reduce the money you spend on health care, the time you spend at the doctor's office, and the time taken away from your family later in life as a result of inactivity. No, you don't need to join a gym, but you do need to find the time to exercise.

If you exercise at home, it can be hard to be consistent. Let's talk about your home environment for a moment. Do you have a clean, organized house? It certainly puts you more in the mood to exercise. "Cleanliness is next to godliness," my grandmother used to say. And organization is a form of discipline that gets you closer to your goals. If you prefer to stay home to exercise until you lose a few pounds, then you need a place to perform your ritual. It could be your bedroom, the basement, even the living room, if no one is going to be in there to interrupt you. Really, you can exercise anywhere you feel comfortable and free from distractions.

Q: My heart beats so fast when I exercise. Is that okay? Why am I out of breath?

A: I tell my gym members that the best way to know if they are working out hard enough is to take the "talk test." While you are doing aerobic exercise, like walking or cycling, you should be able to talk but not sing. So if you can easily belt out "She'll Be Coming 'Round the Mountain" while you are walking, then you need to pick it up a notch. You might want to learn a few new songs, too!

It's not unusual to be short of breath if you have not worked out in a while. If you are having difficulty breathing while exercising, slow down. Try to find a pace that is comfortable but still a challenge. As you consistently exercise, your ability to breathe will improve. Of course, you should go see your doctor to be sure you have no preexisting medical conditions and to discuss the best way to exercise to avoid any potential danger.

Q: If I just go on a diet and don't exercise, will I still lose weight?

A: Yes, you can lose weight through dieting only, but to maintain that weight loss once the dieting is over, you need to exercise. So why not include it to begin with? Exercise helps your motivation grow, making it harder to fail. The benefit of consistent exercise is that you feel less sluggish and more energized. As that energy level grows, so does your motivation. And as to which diet to choose? They all work to some extent, but you'd better pick one you can stick with for the rest of your life. If you think eating a diet of powdered protein shakes or brown rice and tofu is going to work forever, by all means, have at it. I prefer a bit more variety myself, but you'll learn quickly what type of eating plan is sustainable and what will be unacceptable.

Q : But will I ever have time to relax again if I use up my free time on exercise?

A : Your routine may be to go home every day after work, sit on the couch, put your feet up, munch on a bag of chips, have a beer or a glass of wine, watch TV, or busy yourself in front of a computer screen. The latest findings indicate that spending 23 or more hours a week in front of a screen or sitting in your car can have an overwhelmingly negative impact on your health. The idea of that doesn't relax me at all.

Muscle has memory. Just as your body stores memories of physical movement and learns how to do things (like bike or run), your muscles also store the effects of a sedentary lifestyle. Unless you change up your routine, you are going to stay stuck sitting on that couch, doubling your risk of a heart attack as you mistakenly believe that you are just "relaxing." You are wasting precious time—time to share memories with your family, time to prevent cancers from invading your body, time to get to know and love yourself.

Besides, exercise improves your sense of well-being because it releases feel-good brain chemicals (endorphins) that help ease stress and lighten depression. So you'll feel relaxed if you do exercise you enjoy, particularly if you do it socially.

Q: I get bored easily. How can I stick with anything?

A: At my gym, I have found women stick to exercise better in groups. Our group fitness classes are fun and spontaneous. Physical and mental energies feed off each other. The most popular group class at my gym is Zumba, a dance fitness class that incorporates hip-hop and Latin dance styles—like salsa, merengue, and bachata—with lunges and squats. One member described Zumba as being at a nightclub without the alcohol and the men. Another lady refers to our cardio yoga class as "yoga with a beat." Whatever class you choose, the result is the same: Group exercise offers an opportunity to have fun while getting fit.

It's also a great way to boost your mood. It is social, and, unlike jogging or walking on a treadmill, it doesn't get monotonous. I notice women who dance in group fitness classes all have smiles on their faces amid the sweat dripping down their noses because they are engaged in fun, high-energy workouts. The women in the class are not afraid if they miss a beat or step because movement can be expressed freely in class. My fitness motivators do a great job keeping the pace and the women upbeat. That is what a gym should be about—making its members fit, happy, and addicted to feeling good.

But dancing, and even group activities in general, may not be for everyone. Try finding a workout buddy—one person to work out with or just go for a walk with. Or break your workouts into short sessions—10 minutes in the morning, 10 in the afternoon, and then 10 in the evening.

Varying your workout will also help keep you from getting bored—it's hard to enjoy doing the same thing all of the time.

Changing things up will also make you fitter. When you vary your exercise routine, your body works harder to keep up, your fitness is more well-rounded, and, in that process, you actually burn more calories.

Q: **How can I avoid getting too muscular if I exercise? I don't want to look like a body builder!**

A: Listen, it takes a lot of years and a crazy amount of working out to get to body builder level! Simply lifting weights twice a week, even if you are prone to definition, will never cause you to bulk up. I think the question is, really, are muscles attractive? Once upon a time, it was not desirable for women to have sculpted arm or leg muscles. However, Angela Bassett's lean body in *What's Love Got to Do with It* and First Lady Michelle Obama's toned arms have contributed to the idea that it is acceptable, and even fashionable, to have "guns" if you're a woman. How do you make a gorgeous pair of shoes look even better? Nice-looking calves!

Q: **Can I just tone a few areas and not lose weight? I'm big boned. Plus, my man likes me the way I am! He says I'm P-H-A-T and that's sexy.**

A: This is called a coping mechanism—something to make you feel good about yourself whether it is true or not. We all need this sometimes, but let's not be naive or pretend. You have to be honest now: Do you like the weight you're at? Can you do everything you want to do or does your body size hold you back? I'm not saying curves aren't nice, but there is a point where fat puts you at risk for disease and also keeps you from doing things comfortably and joyfully.

As to just toning one area, there is no such thing as spot reduction. You can't lose weight in one area without losing weight in others. Most women focus on wanting to lose weight around their stomach area. Situps and crunches will strengthen your abdominal muscles, but to lose fat anywhere on your body you need to burn calories through aerobic exercise.

Q : **I don't have the time to spend 2.5 hours a week working out. And even if I did, I couldn't do that much exercise. What am I supposed to do?**

A : When in doubt, remember this: Do something as opposed to nothing. You have to start somewhere. If you can only walk for 5 minutes, then walk 5 minutes today. Tomorrow, try increasing it to 6. It's okay to be where you are right now. The important thing is that you start some kind of exercise and stick with it. You will build your stamina and increase the amount of time you work out. But you can't increase something if you ain't doin' nothin'! Change depends on persistence. But we have to do what works in real life. Most of us want to be fit and look good in our clothes, but very few of us are or do. As my father used to say, "A lot of people want to go to heaven, but no one wants to die to get there."

Q : **Okay, I get it! So now what do I do?**

A : Get started by making your own Shape Up Sisters contract with yourself! A contract with yourself can help you set those goals and break bad habits, even when you are feeling full of excuses. As I told the 2,500 participants who signed up for the Shape Up Vicksburg challenge, "You are the most important person in this challenge. It is up to you to decide if you want to commit. It is up to you to decide if you want this for yourself. I can tell you all day that you need to lose weight, exercise, or stop eating this or that, but at the end of the day, the decision is yours. This contract is solely with yourself, and ultimately the only punishments and rewards to be found are within you."

For some people, the prospect of letting themselves down was the hardest thing to deal with. I reminded them that if they got off track . . . so what? At any moment they could get back on track and try again. I suggested that everyone take the contract home and put it on the refrigerator as a reminder to live up to the challenge they set for themselves. "Keep it in plain view, where you can see it clearly each day," I told people. "It should serve as a sign of encouragement to not give up. Hang it visibly on a wall beside your bed, your bathroom mirror, or your refrigerator."

What else to do? Keep reading! The rest of this book is aimed at giving you all the tools you need to succeed.

Shape Up Sisters!
Wellness Contract

I, _____
am aware that this contract is a 90–day commitment to begin a journey to good health and well-being. **I agree to seek progress, not perfection.** I understand small changes toward improving my diet and exercise choices can help me reach my goals.

I understand that hunger, deprivation, and lack of physical activity will not help me on the journey to good health and well-being. Choices to exercise my body and nourish it with healthy foods are ones that can lead to a longer and healthier life.

I commit to improving my lifestyle choices with the three goals I have listed below.

My three short-term goals are:

1. _____
_____
2. _____
_____
3. _____
_____

My three reasons for wanting to do this are:

1. _____
_____
2. _____
_____
3. _____
_____

I will check in with myself daily to explore why my goals are important to me.

Signature: _____ Date: _____

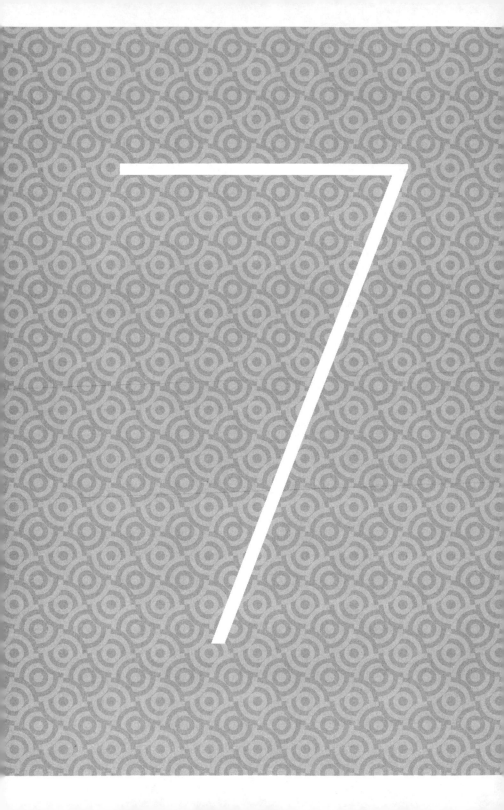

God Don't Like Ugly

Banishing Negativity and Getting Centered

AS MY MAMA LIZA USED TO SAY, "GOD DON'T like ugly." Our thoughts make us who we are, and sometimes thoughts can be ugly. How many of us are in the habit of getting up in the morning and saying, "I will exercise for 30 minutes today"? Yep, that's what I thought!

We tote around a lot of negative assumptions. Instead we think, *I can't exercise today. I'm too busy, too old, too tired, too broke, too fat.* Too many of us focus on the "can't" rather than on the "want," such as, *I want to have fun today. I want to feel good. I want to feel alive in my body.*

One of the things I love so much about my daughter, Chris, is that she doesn't give a hoot about how she looks when she has things to get done. She just jumps right in. She doesn't think, "Do I look right?" or "What will other people think?" Somewhere along the line—I hope it was from me!—she learned that true beauty is opening yourself up to life. Beauty is being able to chase a toddler around your yard. Beauty is dancing with your man. Beauty is shooting some hoops with your teenage son. Beauty is going for a long walk with your best girlfriend and getting to share your feelings with her and make her laugh. Having fun and enjoying life is about loving who you are on the inside and being present in your life. This kind of true beauty comes from letting go of ugliness.

Ugliness is just another way to say *negativity*, in all its forms. Negative words are an obstacle to exercise and really to just about anything you want to do or be in life. Want to ruin a perfectly good day? Be negative. Want to stop short of your full potential? Be negative. Using negative words tells other people a lot about who you think you are and the way you think about the world. Are you a complainer? Are you a victim of everything and everyone? Do you regularly say, "I can't do that" or "I was born this way"?

Negative words are like a vacuum, sucking all the energy out of life. Ask yourself this question: Do I want to be the one who drags my own life down? Of course not. We don't mean to be negative on purpose. Words slip out through mindlessness—your brain on automatic pilot. The more negative words you pile on, the more you fuel negative emotions and the higher the flame burns.

Taking control of your body starts with taking control of your mind. And the first step in that direction is taking control of the words you use and how you use them. In order to create a sustainable program for change, negativity has to be evicted. But for right now, just do this: Make a choice to be positive today. If you make this choice again and again, eventually, it will completely change your life. But just start with right now, today: Every time you start to use a negative word, rephrase it positively.

Can't becomes **Can**

Won't becomes **Will**

But becomes **And**

Shouldn't becomes **Should**

Couldn't becomes **Could**

It might feel a little ridiculous at first. Just go with it. Even if it feels fake, and even if you don't believe right now that **you can** and **you will** and **you should** and **you could,** the words will create a positive change.

Next, change the channel. Most people do not watch television without changing the channel numerous times. You have seen one program, so you flip to the next. You don't want to watch that commercial, so you fast-forward or mute it. You can do the same with negative thoughts. When they come into your mind, change the channel and select a positive one. If the signal isn't coming through clearly, at least tune into a neutral or less-negative channel. Once you have started to get a handle on the words you are using, you are ready to move on and use a technique that will center your thoughts and calm your spirit. You are ready for something that will truly strengthen your relationship with yourself, something that will return your mind to the openness and wonder of a child's mind, something that will make you aware of yourself at a deeper level.

You are ready to meditate.

"Meditate? Huh? What's that?" you might ask.

It is a technique for being quiet.

"Sounds like praying!" you might say.

Don't worry, you are not forsaking your religion. Meditation is where you awaken your Mother Wit, your mental power. It is where you find the indwelling God, the one that speaks to you and answers your prayers. It is where you find the power to stay open to new ideas and have the innocent curiosity of a child. Just by being open to the concept of meditation, you have already started being open to possibility. Meditation isn't weird. You might already have stumbled upon it yourself.

Let me tell you a little story: When I was a young girl, about 10 or so, I never wanted to miss Sunday school or church. When I was there, I felt something that lifted me right into the heart of God. I used to stare for long stretches at one spot on a tapestry that depicted Jesus standing at a table with his hands outstretched to his disciples. Reverend Thomas, gyrating up and down the podium, probably thought I was looking at him, but it was that tapestry that had me mesmerized. As I stared at that one spot—a glow around Jesus's head—all the shouting and fainting in Rose Hill Baptist Church faded into the background. At the time, I did not know what encouragement felt like, but in those moments, as I stared at the tapestry, a sense of stillness and a warm feeling of contentment washed over me. I didn't know it then, but I was meditating.

Modern researchers all over the world are validating what ancient wisdom has always advised: the benefits of practicing meditation and prayer. And science has shown that meditation can increase productivity, decrease stress, combat depression, lower risk of heart attack, and even reduce pain. Two important facts you need to know about your body and mind:

- Your mind and body interact to heal each other.
- The contents of your thoughts and emotions can directly and immediately influence your body—and your actions.

Right now you might be thinking, "This is interesting, but what's this got to do with me losing weight and exercising?" As a lot of research into the mind-body connection has shown, there is no diet or exercise program that will stick for the long term if you don't unleash the power of your mind.

I want you to try this yourself for 5 minutes every morning for 1 week. Real change requires that we learn to nourish and nurture ourselves, and meditation will help you focus your thoughts for the day. It can even be the gateway to other paths that we may have never considered before. By following this little 5-minute ritual—using the same sequence each time—you will learn to meditate and relax, and begin to feel the incredible power the mind has to heal the body.

So do this:

- Drink a tall glass of water. Water helps you refresh and refocus the mind.
- Find a quiet place where you will not be bothered, free from interruptions from children, your husband, and your cell phone. (Even the bathroom will work if it's a place where no one will bother you!) Set a timer for 5 minutes so you don't need to check the clock.
- Sit in a straight-backed chair with your feet flat on the floor and your legs uncrossed. You can prop a pillow behind your back to help you sit up straight. Allow your hands to rest in your lap or on your thighs. Relax your shoulders. Keep your head and neck straight.
- Close your eyes.
- Breathe easily and naturally.
- Try not to think of anything in particular. Let go of the events of the day. There is nothing you need to do in these moments but breathe. Let your breathing deepen, long and slow.
- Tell yourself: "Let go, soften, and relax." Repeat this over and over in your mind.
- If your mind wanders, bring your attention back to breathing deeply and repeat, "Let go, soften, and relax."

This will require effort at first, but keep trying. Eventually, you will be successful. The quiet mind is the mind that has the power to solve whatever problems come up.

- After 5 minutes, bring your attention back to the room. Open your eyes with a smile.

Now you are ready to begin affirmations, which help you build a positive mind-set. To do that, stay seated a couple of minutes longer. You are going to have a short dialogue with yourself. No, talking to yourself doesn't make you crazy; it makes you powerful. Self-dialogue is about self-direction and identity.

The only way you can get an answer is to have a question. Your self-dialogue might go something like this:

Who are you? I am the master of me.

What do you believe? I believe in me.

What do you desire?

What would you like to be?

Your answers are your affirmations. Affirmations really do work, because they program the mind to trust your belief. Repeat your affirmations a few times each day. Say them both quietly and out loud and say them slowly and like you mean them. Tell yourself your affirmations while brushing your teeth, taking a shower, sitting at your desk, driving in your car—whatever works for you.

To create your own affirmation, let your heart speak to you in its truest words. Affirmations can be most powerful when we begin by reversing negative thoughts about ourselves. Our beliefs about ourselves are deeply rooted, sometimes because of criticisms from others or because of certain failures that have convinced us that we can't do or be something. When we believe these negatives, we reinforce them ("I am not worthy" or "I will never succeed at losing weight").

So begin with an "I am" statement that describes what you want to be and feel right now (but don't use "I want!"

because the point is to feel that you *are*). Be positive (so "I am full of energy" rather than "I don't feel tired"). Keep your affirmation simple and in the present ("I am healing" or "I am free from cigarettes"). End by stating your intention for the day: "Today I will make time for myself." Most of all, stay true to what you really feel and want to be, not what you think you should be saying, because those affirmations will have the most power to change your attitude.

Even if you have never meditated or used affirmations before, or you are convinced that it's all just strange, you can do this and benefit from it. If you do it for just a few minutes every day, you will begin to notice positive shifts happening in your life, you will become more aware of your statements and actions, and in the weeks to come you will learn to handle things in your life more responsibly and with grace.

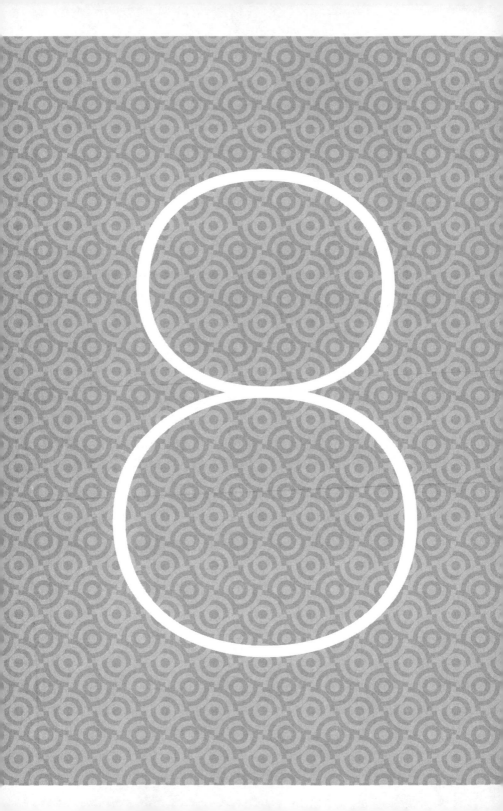

A Closed Mouth Don't Get Fed

Fulfilling Your Needs with Conscious Action, Not Food

H ERE'S SOMETHING WE SAY IN MISSISSIPPI: "A closed mouth don't get fed."

This phrase really encapsulates a philosophy to live by: If you don't speak up about your needs, you don't get what you truly want out of your life. This is a principle that has helped me to achieve what I have today.

At the same time, you could also take this saying to mean, "You are overweight because you eat too much." Here in the South, where it is a cultural belief that a chubby child is a healthy child, we are drawn to the flavor and emotional comfort of the food (and of course we pay attention to the price) before we think about eating to promote good health. We snack, we nibble, we graze, we chow down. Our portions are too big. We don't even know how to eat a meal without over-indulging. And if we aren't eating, we are thinking about eating. So the question is, why do we eat so much? And the answer to this speaks to the other meaning of the saying.

Many of us take refuge in food. We eat not because our stomachs are hungry, but because our souls are hungry. We are lonely, we are bored, we are scared, we are disappointed in ourselves, and so we indulge, comfort, and entertain ourselves with eating. We run around putting other people's needs before our own, and then we are left with nothing to give ourselves but a bag of Fritos and a Big Gulp. We are starving ourselves spiritually and poisoning ourselves physically. But why? What is the hole we are trying to fill with pie and cheeseburgers? Uncovering this hole relates back to the deepest meaning of "a closed mouth don't get fed." If you are not conscious of what is going on inside of you, if you are not aware of your real needs—and, in particular, if you don't speak out about them—how will they ever be fulfilled?

This is true for all of us who really want to manifest change in our lives. You probably think you know yourself pretty well, and you may. If you have a headache, you probably take a couple of aspirin to get rid of the pain, and before you know it the headache is gone. But did you even think to seek out the cause—what might really be bringing on those migraines or throbbing temples? We generate health from within ourselves—and we hinder it, too. When we abuse our body with overeating, overdrinking, overpartying, and lack of sleep, we cause confusion, insecurity, and even illness—and in that state we attract more of the same, rather than attracting what we desire.

Eating should be a conscious and mindful act. One of the easiest ways to curb the amount you eat is to be more aware of your eating habits and why you're eating the way you do. Many of us munch in front of the TV, grab a bite in the car, or get a snack from the vending machine with no regard for whether we are full or even hungry in the first place. And if you think all those "little bites" don't matter, think again. They do.

The biggest obstacles to healthy eating and exercise are the automatic habits that we have fallen into over the years—many of which we're not even aware of anymore. Do you:

- Eat too fast?
- Always clean your plate?
- Eat when you're not hungry?
- Always eat dessert?
- Skip meals (or maybe just breakfast)?

If you don't know the answers to some or all of these, that's a clue that you are running on automatic pilot and aren't being conscious of your actions or your environment. Some habits are good, like always eating breakfast, and some are bad, like always cleaning your plate and having seconds. Some of our habits come from our childhoods and the cultures in which we grew up. But there is an old Bible verse that goes "When I became an adult, I put away childish things." It is never too late to change a habit, no matter how long it has been in your life. The way you do this is by becoming mindful of it and replacing it with a positive behavior.

You need to understand what's eating *at* you so you can change the way you eat. Change requires a thoughtful approach. Check in with yourself before you start to eat: Are you really hungry or are you automatically reaching for a snack? Is there something going on underneath the surface that you feel will be comforted or made right by food? Are you eating simply because it's there? If you are mindful and take a moment to ask yourself these questions, you can start to tune in to what is truly hunger and what is just habit.

The meditation and affirmation rituals that I discussed in the previous chapter—as well as the exercises to become aware of negative language—all go a long way toward helping you become more conscious of your surroundings and more mindful of your actions. There are a few other specific exercises I use to keep myself sharp and conscious of what I'm doing and choosing in the present moment. Try to make some—or all—of these your own practice.

Power of Awareness Exercises

- When you enter a room for the first time, shut your eyes for a second. See how many objects in the room you can name (tables, chairs, desk, pictures, etc.).
- After going up or down a flight of stairs, recall how many there were.
- Think of what you did when you first left the house. What did you do after breakfast?
- As you get ready for bed, try to remember elements of your day. How far did you walk? What did you read? Who did you talk to? Could you have been more polite or shown a little more compassion?

Practice these exercises every day for 3 weeks, or design your own based on your daily routine. For example, reflect on the details as you go to work, take your child to school, or clean your house. They will help you to understand what it means to be aware of your actions, and you will also gain insight into your habits—good and bad—along the way. When you are aware, you can begin to identify the cues in your environment that trigger old habits. For example, if you sit down on the couch, do you always want a bag of potato chips to keep you company? Once you are aware, you can make a different choice, like sitting in a chair and choosing to drink a refreshing glass of ice water, instead. Does having the cookie jar on the counter make you grab a couple as you go by? Put them high up on a shelf or in a cabinet where you—and the kids!—won't see them and be tempted all the time to mindlessly stuff a sugary snack into your mouth.

The next step is training your concentration. You may say, "I don't need to train to concentrate! I can concentrate whenever I want." I can't argue with you about your abilities, but trust me when I say that *everybody* can benefit from a little mental workout. Call me old school, but our reliance on computers and smartphones has made us lazy about exercising our mental sharpness. Tasks that require our brains to focus strengthen our concentration, just like situps strengthen our stomachs. See what I mean by trying these exercises once a day.

Concentration Exercises

- Multiply two two-digit numbers—such as 22 and 28—in your head, without your smartphone. Do it until you are sure the answer is correct.
- Memorize some lines of a poem. For example, here's part of a lovely old poem, "She Walks in Beauty," by Lord Byron:

  > She walks in beauty, like the night
  > 'Of cloudless climes and starry skies;
  > And all that's best of dark and bright
  > Meet in her aspect and her eyes

- When passing a person in a store or on the street, look that person in the face, then look away. Hold that face in your mind for 1 minute. Recall the features of that face. Seek to understand its owner. Did you see fear, pity, joy, sadness, anger? This exercise can be very rewarding because it also teaches you to build more compassion for others.

You won't need to do these forever, but a little practice with them for 3 weeks will give you more control over your thoughts. And gaining control will help you get a grip on that monster that chases all of us at some time or another: *stress*. Stress is one of the most common reasons that we abandon our diet and exercise plans. Stress depletes our self-control and brings on anger and sadness.

It also keeps us fat. A number of studies have shown that stress makes you crave carbohydrate-rich foods—potato chips, pie, cookies . . . you know what I'm talking about. These foods act like a drug that calms your stress hormones. Now, that doesn't mean a Little Debbie Honey Bun is the only thing that will calm you down—heavens, no! An apple and a walk around the block will do it, too. Stress also causes our bodies to store fat. So if you want to get a handle on your weight, you have to make time to relieve that stress buildup.

In the previous chapter, we talked about the importance of affirmations—a form of self-dialogue—to building confidence and feeling good about yourself. But affirmations can also reduce stress and help you turn a negative situation into a positive. Let's say there is a problem that has you feeling confused, hopeless, or discouraged—say, about financial troubles, weight loss, or family conflict. Sometimes it may seem like there is no solution. The ugly thoughts you create and believe not only affect you in the form of stress, but they can also affect others around you. Have a conversation with yourself and then listen for the (true) answer. We often look to other people, places, and things for answers, but in truth, the answers we need are within ourselves. This self-dialogue has you answering only to yourself. Your self-dialogue may go something like this:

How can I solve this problem?
By understanding it.

How can I understand it?
By not fearing it.

How is that accomplished?
By refusing to give it false power over me.

How do I do that?
By seeking more self-knowledge.

Make this dialogue your own by digging deep and asking yourself questions to draw out what's really eating at you and by verbalizing how you *want* to feel, not reflecting back on how you have been feeling. We have already talked about how negative thoughts produce negative results. Ugly thoughts become ugly tendencies. We need to combat negative moods and stress, and the ways we can do this are all around us.

- Listening to music
- Enjoying a cup of tea
- Reading a good book
- Watching a funny movie
- Practicing breath control and meditation
- Exercising—you knew I'd get there again! But truly, if you get hooked on exercise, you conquer many barriers that have kept you down both physically and mentally.
- The power of exercise is well documented, but if you want immediate proof, I recommend taking the time to exercise and looking around at the people who exercise regularly. Are they stronger, can they walk farther, does their skin glow with health? There is all the proof you need.

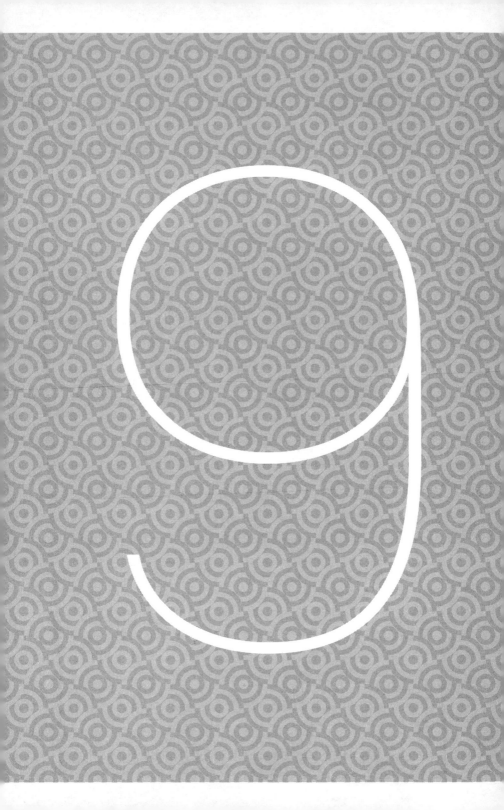

Self-Preservation Is the First Law of Nature

Doing What You Need to Do to Care for Yourself

SOMETIMES I THINK BACK ON MY LIFE AND wonder, "Where would I be today if I had let other people decide what I was to be, instead of what I felt I wanted to be?" My grandmother taught me that self-preservation was about keeping myself alive not just in body, but also in spirit.

As a child, I had to make a lot of adult decisions to stay alive.

One cold morning toward the end of March at age 14, I woke up telling myself to look for a job. I had spent too much of my time making myself available to my boyfriend and not going to work when I should have. The house had a chill and I was not feeling spry, so I pulled the covers over my head to stay in bed a little longer. Then, feeling hungry, I dragged myself from the bed and searched the kitchen for something to eat. As usual, there was no bread. I put on my clothes, feeling irritated about no food ever being in the house. Without washing my face, I picked my Afro, grabbed a coat, and walked the short distance up the hill to the A&P market to steal a loaf of bread.

Standing in the checkout line with the bread concealed nicely under my coat, I began to feel faint. My clever plan, as always, was to pay for a piece of candy or something small so I wouldn't be noticed coming and going out of the store without buying something. Feeling weaker, I thought about leaving, but now I was next in line. Anxious for the cashier to hurry up, I put the Three Musketeers and my quarter on the counter. I pulled my coat closer, leaned on the counter and fainted. The next thing I recall were hands shaking me and a woman's voice making me come around. She was kneeling over me asking, "Honey, are you all right?" I found out later I was 3 months pregnant.

From then on, it was my grandmother who instilled in me that quote I live by today: "Self-preservation is the first law of nature." It sounds selfish and egotistical to some people's ears, I know, but not to mine. You know the safety advice given to anyone with a child on an airplane—how they tell you if there's an emergency to put the oxygen mask on yourself first before you try to help your child? Why do they say that? Because you can't help them if you're incapacitated.

Consider this advice. Putting your own needs first at times like this is crucial. It isn't a selfish act—it's a necessary one.

If *you* do not protect you, then who will? Be true to yourself. It is one of the biggest keys to happiness.

But before I start talking about how our own physical and emotional states affect our families (I'll get to that in the next chapter), I want to encourage you to think about your own needs. We women are caretakers by nature—we stretch ourselves to the limit looking after kids and spouses and aging parents, making sure everyone has what they need, being there for friends or coworkers in a crisis. But who is taking care of the caretaker? Often it's no one, that's who. And though we do deserve support and nurturing from others, we know how hard it can be to ask for it. Instead of taking care of ourselves first, we run around putting other people's needs before our own, starving ourselves spiritually and poisoning ourselves physically.

Here are a few simple steps you can incorporate into your everyday life that will help ensure you are taking care of yourself—in small and not-so-small ways. Watch how much more positive and capable you feel when you do them regularly; that positivity will affect those around you as well.

Self-Care Building Blocks

1. **Start off clean.** Sometimes people roll their eyes when I tell them to approach the day with a clean body. But just the small act of taking a shower and washing off yesterday's problems can help you feel better about yourself.

2. **Wear something nice.** Remember when your mother told you to wear clean underwear with no holes because God forbid you fall down? When you

put on an outfit that you like, you boost your self-confidence. Sure, wearing your pj's to the store may be comfortable and convenient, but you'll stand up a little straighter if you feel that you look presentable. A blouse that is clean and neat reflects a side of you—the polished, poised, "I got this" side—that you want people to see.

3. **Appreciate yourself.** How do you view yourself? When you look in the mirror, do you see beauty? Do you focus on all the so-called negative aspects of your appearance? You have the power to view yourself any way you'd like, and the way you view yourself is directly related to your self-confidence. So when you look at yourself and you recognize your beautiful smile, your bold forehead, and your soulful eyes, then this is what you will reflect to other people. Smile when you are driving in your car; someone is looking.

4. **Use gratitude to change your attitude!** When we are grateful, we are humble. Even with a plateful of problems, we can all find something to appreciate. Just as focusing on solutions rather than problems helps you feel more confident, choosing to see the blessings in your life rather than the hardships helps you feel more grateful. Acknowledge your struggles, but be equally grateful for your strengths.

5. **Fake it until you make it.** Smile even when you don't feel like it. When you don't feel like being positive, act as if you are anyway. Stay with it and you will feel a little happier. Also, people are attracted to others with positive attitudes and they will appreciate that quality in you.

6. **Play well with others.** How is this related to well-being? When you treat people nicely, including

yourself, you feel good and believe that you are a good person.

7. **Get prepared.** Sometimes it's hard to feel confident walking into a situation unprepared. We can't prepare for everything, but in those times when you can take steps to be ready for a situation, do it. For example, are you interviewing for a job? Find out at least one thing about the place where you're applying and the person you're meeting with. The Internet is a wonderful thing! When you go into a situation feeling prepared, your self-confidence rises, too.

8. **Add some color to your to-do list.** What have you been meaning to do, week after week, that you keep putting off? Get out your list of tasks and goals and take action on one of the items. Then cross it out in red ink. As you knock them off, one by one, you'll feel the progress and will be inspired to do more. Procrastination damages self-confidence.

9. **Give for a cause.** You gave at church and you are smiling! Now offer help to someone else. When we help others, we feel better about ourselves. One study shows that lending a sympathetic ear and being there for your friends actually reduces the risk of heart attack, and another study found that those with chronic pain reported a reduction in pain when they reached out to others who were also suffering. Find a cause or an issue that inspires you and offer to help. Do you like what you are reading in this book? Great! Now think about how gratifying it would be to help someone else who is struggling. Buy them this book. Even just telling them what you've learned and listening to them gives them the gift of your attention. We all have gifts to offer, and they don't have to be material things or cost money. Choose an act of kindness and do it.

10. **Stand like a mountain.** Your posture can greatly affect your self-confidence. When you slouch or lean to one side all the time, you are projecting a sense of weakness. Pull your head up and your shoulders back. As your body holds this strong stance, it gives you confidence. The next time you are at the store or some public place, notice how people stand. Which people look more confident? More attractive?

11. **Educate yourself.** Knowledge is power, regardless of whether it is self-knowledge, career knowledge, religious knowledge, or any other knowledge. When you are educated, you feel more competent. You don't have to know everything, but find things in your life that you like or want to know more about, and then Google them or ask other people their opinions—or even try the old-school way of just going to the public library! Empower yourself with knowledge.

12. **Work on your goals.** I define a goal as something that challenges you just enough that you believe you can achieve it. (To lose 5 pounds in a month is achievable, but 30 pounds in a month is a fantasy.) Start off with a goal that is attainable. Achieve one small goal, then another, and slowly you will build confidence in yourself. As your confidence grows, you can increase the difficulty of your goals.

13. **Shift your attention from problems to solutions.** We have a tendency to obsess about our problems, giving them a life of their own. Try overpowering problems with solutions. If you have money worries, ask yourself how you can start to save money. Even a slight shift in thinking can create

results (and savings). When you are solution-based and open to ideas for how to change a situation, you will feel more confident and be more likely to succeed.

14. **Let the snow globe settle.** Sometimes life is chaotic and messy. When you can, let the pieces fall so you can get your bearings and make good decisions. Take time to sit quietly and let your mind and body reset. Having space to breathe is very important. When we are overwhelmed by chaos, we do not feel confident or effective. Five minutes of quiet time at the beginning of each day can do wonders for your well-being. You can focus on breathing, prayer, or meditation, or you can just lie down with your eyes closed. Your brain will appreciate this time and reward you for it.

These simple steps can help you focus on meeting your needs and set you on the path to a more productive, confident life. You need to be committed to you. When you have confidence, it is hard to be negative and easy to see possibilities. Even if yours is shaky right now, "Fake it 'til you make it" should be your mantra.

This confident mind-set is so important for us women, who typically are the caretakers, grocery shoppers, cooks, and role models of the family. Only *you* have the right to determine who you are. Every day say to yourself, "Today I will be a role model and I will respect myself." Just starting there is empowering and a change for the better. Self-respect begets respect from others.

You already know it's true. Now go live it, Sister.

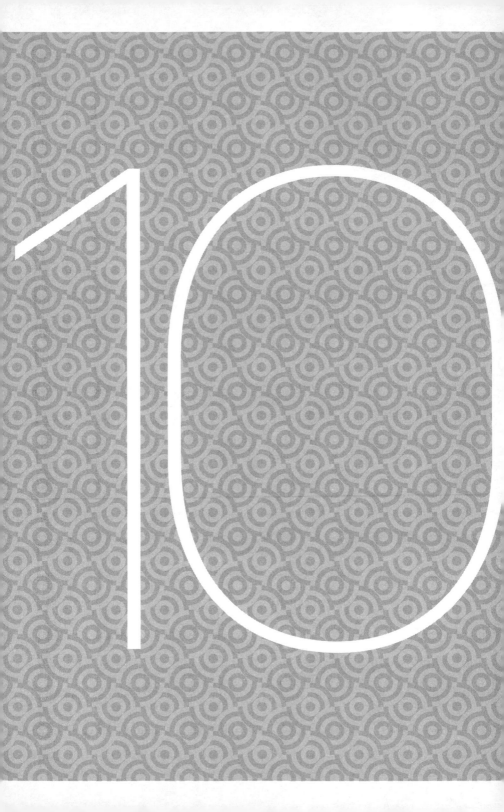

The Family That Plays Together

Getting the Support of Your Family

YOU KNOW THE SAYING "WHEN MAMA'S NOT happy, nobody's happy"? That's right. You are the center of your family, whether you know it or not. And when you make a change, even if it's for the better, it's going to cause ripples. Sometimes it will even cause resistance. The people around you will have to consider whether they also need to change, and that can be uncomfortable for them to confront. They may even start to resent, rather than appreciate, what you are trying to do for yourself and for them.

But if you persist, eventually you will get everyone to share in charting the course to a healthier, more vibrant family life. Speak up and never give up.

Let me tell you this from my own life: I have lived with and struggled with the weight-related issues of the people I love as if they were my own. While I have never really struggled with my own weight, I have struggled with the right to stay healthy.

I am often teased for making healthy choices, like exercising, not drinking soda pop, and eating egg-white omelets.

"You think you're too good to eat a fried bologna sandwich?" they say.

"You're weird," they tell me. They call me a health nut.

I take it all with a grain of salt. Sometimes we mock others because we want to feel good about our bad choices.

Becoming aware of the danger of letting others make decisions for you helps put those kinds of comments into perspective. Constantly ask yourself, "Who is in control?" Sometimes it can be easier to believe we are not in control of ourselves so we can blame others if things aren't going right. But the real answer is this: "*I* am in control."

I have had to fight against the idea that choosing to take care of myself is a selfish act, instead of an act of self-love and self-respect that ultimately benefits everyone around me.

Many of us know how difficult it is to get our companions off the couch and into exercise. Let me tell you, fighting for better health when it's your spouse who has the issue is no easy task. My husband, Jim, is a man who enjoys creature comforts. He's the kind of guy who loves good food, enjoys a beer, and would much rather sit back and soak up the sun than run around in it. At one time, Jim weighed 270 pounds. Being that he is 5 feet 10 inches tall, I worried that all those extra pounds made him a dead man walking, especially since Jim's father had died of a heart attack at age 49.

Trying to get someone you love to lose weight because you don't want them to live with disease or die young is one of the hardest challenges to face. For a long time, Jim wasn't even willing to try new, healthy foods that I would introduce at home. "Linda, I don't want to eat cardboard!" he would bellow, assuming that all healthy food did not taste good.

Exercise was no easier. For years I woke up at 5:30 a.m. to work out just because Jim didn't want our morning routine to change. He wanted to relax, have coffee, and read the newspaper together, just like we had always done. After a couple years of this, I had the bright idea that if I could get him to join me for a workout in the comfort of our own home, I could organize my time better and motivate him to exercise.

We started out with an easy video by Leslie Sansone called *Walk Away the Pounds*. I imagined we would start by walking 1 mile, work up to 2 miles, then 3 miles, over several months. Well, it took Jim more than a year to make it past 1 mile, and he never committed to three times a week. Scratch that idea.

Next we got him a personal trainer at a gym. Guess what? Jim chitchatted his way through most of those workouts. I don't think he even broke a sweat most of the time.

He would say he was doing Weight Watchers; he would try the Atkins diet—until he wanted an ice cream, and then all bets were off. I consulted Jim's son, who is a medical doctor, about what options we had to help his dad. He recommended gastric bypass surgery. That did help initially, but because Jim didn't change his behaviors, the weight came back.

Sometimes we would argue about it. I tried to avoid shutting down when I ran up against his resistance to change. Sometimes, through talking it out, understanding would start to creep through his stubbornness, and sometimes I could even understand his side of the argument. But I never gave up trying to change his unhealthy habits, even if we fought. This was an urgent cause for me. If Jim continued down this road, I knew his destination.

"You want me to end up a rich widow?" I asked him.

"All right, all right," he said. "I'll try the gym again."

Today, thanks to help from his trainer, Alvin Stimage, whose focus and skill helped get Jim on track with workouts at the YMCA 5 days a week, Jim now weighs 200 pounds. Now he feels much better and walks with me for the enjoyment of it—and generally has a more active lifestyle. There's no argument anymore! Best of all, his doctor—otherwise known as his son, Dr. Fondren!—has given him a clean bill of health.

It's hard to be the health crusader when the cards seem stacked against you. My sisters Pat and Martha, like my sister Mary who died, have battled obesity. I struggled with finding ways to make my own decisions, knowing that I, too, could easily fall into overeating. For as much as I know now about diet and exercise, it is not all about *knowing*. It's about faith, taking a chance on change . . . whatever you want to call it.

It's also about doing. And it's often difficult to do what you know is right when circumstances, and people in your life, aren't supportive. Sometimes I want a light dinner, but we are invited to a dinner party. Sometimes I want to go for a walk and Jim wants to see a movie. Like every woman, I am challenged to balance time, money, husband, family members, Facebook, friends, cooking, shopping, driving children or grandchildren around, and dealing with issues at work. Making choices each day is a constant experiment in mind control that always comes back to this question: How much am I worth to myself?

Do this: Get out a photo of yourself from when you were a child. Look at the photo. Would you say to yourself as a child, "You are not worth taking care of"? Of course not. But, in fact, that is exactly what you are saying to yourself today when you do not make healthy choices.

How you answer that question of worth ripples out to your family, especially to your children. Anyone with kids knows that they watch us for signals of how to act. If they see us making unhealthful choices that are harmful to our well-being, then they will make those choices, too. When we decide to change ourselves, we are changing our children, too. If you model healthy habits, your kids will take the cue and follow your lead.

The women at my gym remind me every day by sharing their stories and anxieties that obesity is crippling the very foundation of our families. One-third of all children in this country are overweight or obese, according to a number of studies. The Robert Wood Johnson Foundation estimates that roughly 23 million American children and adolescents are overweight or obese and that black and Mexican American children ages 2 to 19 are more overweight than white children in the same age group. The foundation's research also shows that obese teens have roughly an 80 percent chance of becoming obese adults. And obese adults are more likely to have higher medical expenses and ultimately live a shorter life.

This problem is not all on you. Many factors are at work. Our food environment makes it very hard for us to make good choices. We are constantly being shown pictures of glistening desserts and juicy triple-decker burgers. Advertising is so realistic that we can practically smell the french fries just from looking at a picture in a magazine. It's powerful stuff. Vending machines and convenience stores are on nearly every corner, and they rarely, if ever, carry any food that could be considered healthy.

You may not have caused the problem, but you are a big part of the *solution.* We women are still in charge when it comes to making decisions for how our families are living and eating. If a mother is overweight, chances are her entire family is overweight, as well. It will be difficult for you to start a healthy lifestyle if your husband and children are not a part of it. The success rate is so much higher when a family works together.

Let's take that old adage "The family that prays together, stays together" and make one change: "The family that *plays* together, stays together." Children love to move, and the more you turn moving into play, the more fun and success you will all have. The Physical Activity Guidelines for Americans advises that children and adolescents should do 60 minutes (1 hour) or more of physical activity daily. Be sure to include vigorous aerobic activity on at least 3 of those days. Running, walking, jumping rope, and playing on the monkey bars are all good ways of getting that level of activity. Go out for a bike ride together. Visit the community pool or local basketball court. Try skipping races, throw a Frisbee, play freeze tag. Don't have bikes or pool access? Put on some thumping music in the living room, push the furniture out of the way, and create a home disco. Strike up a dance. Let them move their bodies in all sorts of ways. Add arm flares, leg jerks, and hip action. Music helps move the spirit. Your kids will love it, and so will you.

Make moving part of family life. Not only will it bring you closer together, it will establish healthy habits that your kids will someday hand down to their own kids. I can already hear you say, "How do I drag them away from TV and video games?" Well, you turn off the TV. Yes, it is that simple. They might scream and yell for a while, but ask yourself how they got that habit. At the deepest level, children desire to be with us and they want our attention. They will follow your lead, if you take it often enough.

Shopping together is a great opportunity to get your kids involved in healthy eating habits. In Part 3, I will show you how to read the nutritional information on food labels. Show your kids what you have learned and put them on the lookout for added chemicals, corn syrup, and calories. Teach them how to pick out a ripe melon or a crispy head of lettuce. Give them their own shopping list and let them fill their own cart. It will give them a sense of ownership with food choices. Let children experience for themselves what you are telling them—they will learn better when they are hands-on.

Little kids love to help in the kitchen. Hand them a bunch of carrots and a peeler and let them go. They *want* to shuck the corn or rinse berries in a colander. This is play to them, and playing is learning. Let your home be a laboratory for healthy living. They will carry what they learn from you about food and fun throughout their lives.

You can also encourage healthy competition and make a chart for your family using the gold star system: Every time anyone in the family eats a vegetable or a fruit at dinner, put a gold star on the chart. Have a reward system for when a certain number is obtained.

Teachers can tell students all the reasons they need to eat fresh vegetables. But at the end of the day, what they learn about healthy eating comes back to what they find at home in the refrigerator and in the cupboards. As parents or grandparents, we need to be vigilant. Children do not own the decision to put unhealthy foods in their bodies. Parents and adults need to be accountable for those actions.

In 2005, 43 percent of Mississippi's elementary school students were obese or overweight. By 2011 thanks, in part, to the leaders across Mississippi working together to create a new culture of health that promotes regular physical activity and healthy eating in our schools, those rates have dropped to 37.3 percent, according to the Robert Wood Johnson Foundation. Another important factor has been the Let's Move! initiative launched by First Lady Michelle Obama, dedicated to solving the problem of childhood obesity. These efforts recognize that by giving kids balanced meals; eliminating added sugars; and offering fresh vegetables, fresh fruits, and whole grains, they are fueled up for better learning. The state act even aims to eliminate fried foods—a staple in Mississippi—from school meals. Unfortunately the adult obesity rate is more entrenched, but I have made it my mission, as you know, to change that, too.

Sometimes it might be easier to eat carelessly when we are pressed for time or just pick up fast food when we are rushing home from work, but these quick decisions directly affect the future of our children and the habits they carry into adulthood. I know it's fashionable to say how bad fast-food restaurants are, but I go to McDonald's myself. It's unrealistic to say we won't go, especially when parents have easy access to fast-food joints in every neighborhood. But that doesn't mean we can throw caution to the wind and eat a double cheeseburger and fries. Most places now have low-cal options, such as salads, wraps, apple slices, and low-fat milk. I know kids want junk, but instead of giving in, buy the toy separate from the meal if you want to give them a treat. This way you teach them that good choices come with a reward, too.

Reversing the statistics can't be done by the government or legislators alone; we are our children's first teachers—both in the home and in our communities.

My work with children is very important to me. For a Rotary Club–sponsored literacy project, I took on the job of delivering dictionaries to classrooms at a local elementary school. This was after I had been nominated as a CNN Hero. Kids in town often refer to me as "Ms. Fondren, the hero lady." We looked up different words during my visit, and I showed them through my actions what it means to be of service. After I left, one student told the principal, "I would like to come in early in the mornings to help pick up around the school."

The principal returned the request with a nod and said, "That's very good." As the boy was walking away, she asked him, "Why? Why do you want to do that now?"

He replied, "That hero lady came to class and told us we have to be of service to everybody. So I want you to know I want to come in early and help." That was the cutest thing. At a young age, this boy understood what it means to be of service. I hope this lesson will continue with him far beyond the classroom and help guide him in his decisions.

I also volunteer with the Vicksburg Warren School District's nutrition director, Gail Kavanaugh, and together we lead a student activity called Fun Fitness Friday. She teaches the students about basic nutrition and I give them fun exercises to do. At first, the students can be apprehensive, especially the younger ones, because they're not sure why they are there. But when I jump in with the fitness fun that gets them pumped up, the little girls and boys can't help but jump up with me. I absolutely love the happy, excited expressions on their faces. At this moment, I see their innocence. They do not care about what we, as adults and parents, have to go through, like paying bills or getting to work on time. They just want to have fun and the attention of someone they look up to.

One afternoon, a pair of really sharp twin boys in the third grade wanted to show me their dance moves. One was so excited to show off his Michael Jackson moonwalk, which he had been working on. While he was demonstrating, a small crowd of his classmates formed around him, cheering him on. I gave him a big smile and clapped. That was all he needed at that moment—a little bit of appreciation to boost his self-esteem. After our fitness session was over, he ran over to me and gave me an enormous hug and a huge smile. He said, "Thank you, ma'am."

That gesture had an enormous impact on me. It felt absolutely fantastic. It reminded me that the gift of our attention is free and is just about the greatest way we can nourish each other's well-being.

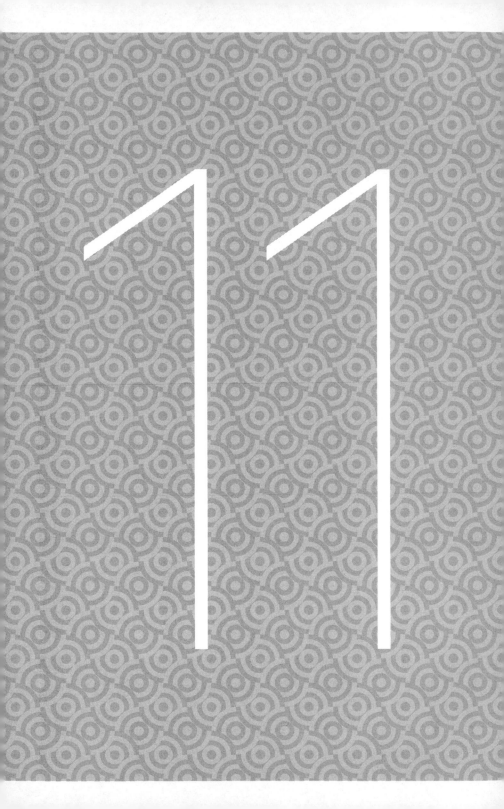

Move It to Lose It

Finding Ways to Fit In Exercise

I F THERE IS A CORE VALUE IN MY LIFE, AND IN MY message, it is to dream big, but start small. No doubt some of you, like some Vicksburg residents, have a lot of weight to lose—maybe more than 100 pounds. But if you take on the whole problem at once, you will defeat yourself before you have even begun. There's an old joke that goes, "How do you eat an elephant? One bite at a time."

The cause of obesity has many faces. And, yes, poverty is a factor. But what is overlooked is plain old lack of effort. If we want something bad enough, like losing weight for a wedding or class reunion, we put in the effort. Once we make it, we go back to the old comfort zone. This has always been a big challenge for me. That is why this chapter is focused on sustained effort.

When a person wants to lose weight, they might immediately start running because that is what they think they are supposed to do. But if they haven't exercised in 3 years, then that is unrealistic. It ends in pulled muscles, exhaustion, and failure. As we've discussed before, you are better served beginning with a small, achievable goal, like walking for 10 minutes each day, and then gradually working up to longer stretches of time. Pretty soon, you might find yourself breaking up that walk with a light jog. Perhaps you'll even end up running, but it doesn't matter if you run, because you're already exercising. You've achieved your small goal.

Yeah, maybe showing up at your high school reunion in a size 12 dress is your short-term goal. But your long-term goal is sustained weight loss. So go buy that dress and hang it on the closet door to look at and dream on. Don't go beating yourself up because it doesn't fit today. What can you do instead? Eat a raw vegetable, skip dessert, drink a glass of water instead of a soda, go for a walk, or just take a deep, mindful breath. These are simple things that let you win *right now*. They add up, and before you know it, they will be slipping you into that dress anytime you want to wear it.

So try not to tackle the whole problem at once. It's more important to just start somewhere today. Don't say to yourself, "I will never eat dessert again." Of course you will. Just say, "I won't eat dessert right now." Then you can decide what you want to do tomorrow when tomorrow comes. That's how you win. So right now you can make a healthy choice. And that choice is going to make you feel good. It won't make you a size 12 today, but it will make you feel like you are in charge of yourself. And as a bonus, you get to enjoy putting on a smaller dress along the way.

Losing weight and getting healthy is a marathon, not a sprint. In your marathon, instead of feeling exhausted as you approach the finish line, you will feel more energized. You will cross that finish line and find that you want to keep going because you feel so good. That is success.

But like a marathon, every mile counts. You might relate

to Monique. Like clockwork, Monique shows up three times a week to work out for 30 minutes on the treadmill at my gym. She goes through the motions, doing the same lackluster routine. She admits she's on the verge of quitting. Her complaint? "I haven't lost any weight!" Turns out that the only time she moves is those three times a week. Otherwise she is taking the elevator, sitting at a desk for 8 hours, driving home, doing some housework, then collapsing in front of the TV until it's time to do it all over again the next day.

This probably sounds surprising coming from me, since I own a gym, but it's the truth: A gym membership won't do you much good if you don't get in the habit of moving more throughout the day. This habit is free. When you start to move more, you start to change your idea that exercise is something you have to do at a gym. You've got a body; you can move it any minute you choose to.

"Every little helps a little," the saying goes, and little changes in your health add up to big changes. I challenge you to add the following easy exercises to your everyday life, and be sure to include the simple strategies listed after the exercises, as well. You'll be fitter and more able to enjoy life than ever before without even realizing how you did it!

The Gym of Life

Exercises are great, but there are so many other ways to slip in more movement throughout your day. Try some of the following suggestions and think of some of your own!

1. **Stop driving around** the parking lot looking for the spot closest to the entrance. Park at the other end and laugh at everybody else as they jockey for spaces to squeeze into.

2. **After you finish grocery shopping,** take one full lap around the store with your full cart.

3. **Instead of leaving your shopping cart** in the parking lot, take it to the return area. You get a little extra exercise, and your stray cart won't dent any cars!

4. **Don't just return your cart,** look for carts that others have left in the parking lot, too. Do a good deed and burn calories by returning an extra one to the bin.

5. **Rethink fashion:** Wear your tennis shoes as much as possible so you'll be free to walk comfortably and for longer distances.

6. **Pretend that every elevator** and escalator is broken. Take the stairs whenever possible.

7. **While you are talking** on your cell phone, pace around rather than stand in place.

8. **Have to stand in line?** Do 10 calf raises (raising yourself onto the balls of your feet). Something is better than nothing, and who knows, you might inspire other people in line to do the same thing.

9. **Bend over and touch your toes** once for every letter in your name. If your name has four letters or less, then use your last name, too.

10. **Make an agreement** with your children: For every *A* they bring home, you will do five pushups. If you can't do pushups, do situps.

11. **Clean the bathtub.** Bend over and scrub that tub! You'll burn calories and build muscle.

12. **Play "Head, Shoulders, Knees, and Toes."** Sing it and go through the sequence four times during your day—at home, at work, even on vacation. You'll get your blood pumping and benefit from the stretch.

13. **Play tag with your kids.** It burns calories, and the

excitement of being chased gets your endorphins flowing and heart rate pumping.

14. **Shake your groove thang!** Dancing is great exercise and improves mood. So when you are listening to your iPod or watching *Dancing with the Stars*, bust out your inner Beyoncé.

15. **Go for the clean stretch:** When you are in the shower, wash your legs and feet without propping your leg on the side of the tub. Over time, this will help improve flexibility.

16. **Do the toothbrush balancing act.** When you brush your teeth (hopefully twice a day, but I'm no dentist), stand on your right leg and brush the right side of your mouth for 1 minute, then switch legs and brush the left side of your mouth for 1 minute.

17. **Try skipping.** Whether you are with your kids or on your own, skip a little. You'll feel younger and reap the benefits of increasing your heart rate.

18. **Bring in the groceries** by yourself. Instead of calling on your family to help unload the car, take the time to do it on your own. Lift heavy bags by tightening your stomach muscles and using your legs, rather than bending over, to avoid hurting your back.

19. **Plant a garden.** Even a small amount of gardening calms the nerves and engages muscles that we don't use often enough. You can connect with the earth and with yourself.

20. **During TV commercials,** stand up, jog in place, or raise and lower your arms—anything to move your body.

21. **Don't cut corners.** If you are walking somewhere, don't take the shortest route.

22. **Be ambidextrous.** If you are right-handed, try using

your left hand for some of your chores and activities. You will engage both sides of your brain and train your muscles to be more balanced and efficient.

23. **Arm wrestle your kids!** Your arms will become toned and firm, and all the laughter it will cause will exercise your stomach muscles, too.

24. **Try My Bonnie Boogie.** Remember that old song? *"My Bonnie Lies Over the Ocean"*? Grab a kitchen chair, stand in front of it, and sing the song. Every time you sing a word that starts with B, either sit or stand.

25. **Stand up** in your office or cubicle at least once every hour; it burns more calories than sitting!

26. **Roll your shoulders.** Even while you are sitting down, you can slowly curl your shoulders forward 5 times, and circle them back. This relieves tension and improves range of motion.

27. **Drink enough water** so that you have to go to the bathroom frequently, which forces you to get up and walk around.

28. **Be old-fashioned.** Don't use an electric device when a hand tool will do.

29. **Be inefficient.** Don't make one trip by foot when you can make three. Or five.

30. **Get up and get it yourself.** If you are sitting on the couch, don't ask your child or husband to fetch you a snack.

31. **Try engaging in quick bursts of activity:** Jump or skip. You will increase your energy, burn more calories, and feel younger.

32. **Rent a comedy** and don't hold back on the laughter. Laughing strengthens your core muscles and increases the feel-good chemicals in your brain.

33. **Get a step counter or pedometer.** These small tools are cheap and track how much you move. Set a goal of taking 10,000 steps a day. If you only hit 9,000, walk around the house and see if you can't bump up the number.

34. **Wii shall overcome.** Video games are a problem when you or your child just sits on the couch. Try some of the Wii Fit games. They are fun for the whole family and can require a lot of movement.

35. **Fidget.** Research has shown that people who fidget have lower rates of obesity and burn more calories.

36. **Rearrange the furniture.** Try moving that chair to the other side of the room. If you don't like it, move it back. Be careful not to move something too heavy, but don't be afraid to exert yourself.

37. **Try walking prayers.** Often we kneel or sit still when we pray. Go for a prayer walk.

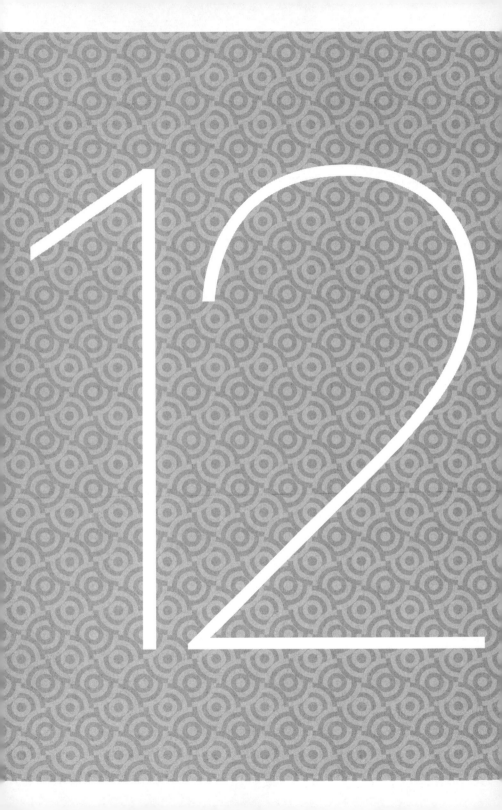

A Stitch in Time Saves Nine

**Planning Strategies for Healthy Eating
on a Budget**

YOU'VE GOT TO LOVE MY SISTER PAT. SHE informed me one day that her cholesterol was over 300 and her blood pressure was 170/90. She had complained about gaining weight over the past year, convincing herself that it was all due to rare medical conditions that she spent hours researching on the Internet. She would look up symptoms and then diagnose herself. Finally I said to her, "Girl, you're looking at every cause but yourself and your choices." But I just could not convince her to look in the mirror to find the problem.

After what seemed like her 100th doctor's visit, Pat finally got the message that her high cholesterol could kill her. "Give me those good diet recipes you use," she told me. "I don't want to have to figure out the calories and fat and things. I want it already done." I wanted to say, "What about all those hours you spent looking up your illnesses?" But I didn't. I just handed over the recipes—some of which I will share with you at the end of this book.

Here's the thing: It's not enough to simply *want* to make positive lifestyle changes, or even to research what it is you want to do. All of your good intentions for improving your habits will crumble if you don't have a plan. The old saying "A stitch in time saves nine" tells us that a little forethought can save us a lot of unneeded effort later. This is why you have got to plan, plan, and then plan some more to overhaul your eating habits. Because if you haven't planned, sooner or later you'll find yourself swinging through a drive-thru saying " . . . and give me fries with that."

Now, "planning" isn't a big deal. It's a recipe or a shopping list. It's having the items you need on hand and stocking up on staples, which can make all the difference when you face your favorite excuse—"lack of time." Planning is getting rid of unhealthy foods in your cupboard. It is taking a moment to sit with your family to discuss bringing back family dinners and setting aside time to eat together at the table, making them aware that taking charge of their health is no joke. Planning is deciding what you're going to get before you step into that supermarket.

Planning is an ongoing activity. This is not something you do once and forget about. New habits take some time to become second nature, just like buying that bag of Cheetos used to be second nature. The difference is, one kind of habit is giving us years of healthy living and enjoying our family's company, and the other is leading us to the hospital and the mortuary.

All good intentions go out the window when we get overwhelmed, so *plan, plan, plan*. Even one of my most experienced instructors at Shape Up Sisters, Trophia Robinson, admits that she must keep herself organized when it comes to eating. "One of my struggles with staying healthy is resisting the temptation of unhealthy foods. It's always difficult to fight the urge for fried chicken with corn bread," Trophia admits with a smile. "Exercise has never been a problem, but keeping a healthy meal plan that goes along with fitness is the true challenge for me."

The way she gets around that challenge is by either bringing a healthy lunch from home, or ordering only the healthy versions of take-out foods (a baked sweet potato instead of a regular one) and carrying around healthy snacks like fruits and nuts that she can snack on every couple of hours instead of reaching for unhealthy treats. Planning will determine your success. You need to stick to a few strategies, though: Rethink old ways of doing things, shop right, think through costs, and know how much you are eating.

How to Shop at the Supermarket

You might be thinking, "What's she talking about? I've been shopping at the supermarket all my life!" Yes, but you may be guessing your way through the aisles, trying to make sense of all the stuff on the shelves. New products advertised as "healthy" and "natural" are constantly showing up in grocery stores. It's hard to know what to believe! But if you prepare a little before you leave, what you serve at your table can be a whole lot healthier, and you'll probably save some money, too. (Studies show that when you have a grocery list you're less likely to give in to impulse purchases.) Remember: What's good for you is good for the whole family. You don't have to buy special foods or cook meals for yourself if all of you eat the same way. Turn the page and get started.

Plot and Plan

Create a shopping list and don't divert from it. According to the Food Marketing Institute, you spend $2 for every minute you are in the grocery store. Plan your meals on a weekly basis and decide what you need for cooking. Planning ahead can save time and money.

Know the layout of the local grocery stores. Usually, you will find the fresh foods that will form the basis of your meals—like fruits and vegetables, meat, fish, chicken, and dairy—in the outer aisles, so put those at the top of your list. The inner aisles are where processed and prepackaged foods are stocked, so put them below the produce, meats, and dairy. This way you can skirt the aisles with the least-healthy temptations. Lots of junk foods—cookies, sugary cereals, and candy—are shelved at your kids' eye level, so be sure to steer clear of these hazards when you shop with your children, unless you are prepared to deal with their meltdowns when they want everything they see.

Fresh Isn't Always Best

The idea that "fresh is best" applies only to those who have access to fresh produce, intend to eat it, and can afford it. And fresh isn't always better in terms of nutritional quality. Fruits and vegetables that are flash-frozen or canned (in water) are an affordable and healthy way to incorporate more fruits and vegetables into your diet. Produce is often picked, washed, and frozen or canned in a short span of time. This process actually helps lock in some of the nutrients that can be lost when produce is transported across the country or sits on a grocery shelf for days. And canned fish packed in water is also a healthy option.

Keep assorted canned and jarred foods on hand so you can always whip up easy, nutrient-packed meals: tomato sauces, tuna, vegetables, beans, and fruits (see page 154 for a list of Better Kitchen Staples for all of these food types).

Vegetables should be canned in water with no added salt, and fruit should be packed in its own juice. If you can't find it packaged this way, put the fruit or veggies in a strainer and rinse off the added syrup or sauce before you eat it.

The frozen food section can be your second-best choice for veggies, like green beans, broccoli, cauliflower, and spinach. Note that frozen vegetables prepared with sauces are often high in sodium, and though they are quick to cook, they aren't the best for your blood pressure or health.

Shop Once a Week

No one "drops by" the grocery store without overspending. In fact, the typical American throws out 40 percent of their food every month, according to the National Resources Defense Council. Save money and avoid food spoilage by purchasing only a week's worth of perishable items. For instance, if you want apples and cheese sticks as a snack for the upcoming week, then purchase five to seven apples and five to seven cheese sticks, no more. (In the next chapter I've got plenty more tips on how to stock your kitchen with simple healthy basics that last.)

Eat Before You Shop

A full stomach will not lead you into temptation! But when you are hungry, everything looks good. If you can't get a meal before you go, munch on an apple and have some water or grab a couple of whole wheat crackers and a tablespoon of peanut butter.

Bulk Buy with Caution

Buying in bulk can save you money on some items, but not all. Purchase pantry staples—such as grains, beans, coffee, and oils—in bulk. Avoid buying large quantities of perishable condiments, dairy items, and unhealthy snacks. Reconsider purchasing large frozen bags of food. Unless it's a true family favorite and a meal staple, these frozen items are often forgotten about, making them a waste of money.

Read It before You Eat It

Knowing how to read a nutrition label will help you make healthier choices.

Nutrition labels tend to be confusing, and many food manufacturers want to keep it that way! But understanding how to read a label and what all of those percentages mean can be empowering and can help you make better decisions. The place to start is the serving size, which is the first piece of information listed on any label. Very important: Notice *how many* servings are in a package or container. If you double the serving size, you double the calories. Around 40 calories per serving is low, while 400 calories a serving is high.

Now, check out the daily value portion of the label. This indicates what percentage of your daily allowance each nutrient represents. For better health, look for foods that contain 5 percent or less of each of the following nutrients. Avoid foods with more than 20 percent of each one. This is simply a quick benchmark to use to help keep your pantry staples within an ideal range for health.

1. **Saturated fat.** Found in animal products, saturated fat (the kind that is solid at room temperature) can increase your risk of heart disease and stroke. Meat and full-fat dairy products, like sausage, butter, and whipped cream, are high in this type of fat.

2. **Trans fats.** These processed fats also increase your risk of heart disease. These are in a lot of packaged foods—they are listed on the ingredients as partially hydrogenated oils—because trans fat extends the shelf life. Everything from meat sticks to frozen pizzas to microwave popcorn and even coffee

creamers have them. Fortunately, the FDA may soon phase trans fats out of processed foods.

3. **Cholesterol.** Like saturated fat, cholesterol is found in animal products only (so fruits and vegetables are cholesterol free). There are good and bad types of cholesterol (and your body produces cholesterol, too), but too much of the bad type of cholesterol (LDL, or low-density lipoproteins) can clog arteries, raising your risk of heart attack and stroke.

4. **Sodium.** Another word for salt, most of the sodium in our diets comes from processed, packaged foods. Too much sodium can increase your risk of high blood pressure. Foods that are particularly high in sodium include breads and rolls, packaged meats, pizza, soups, and sauces.

5. **Sugar.** There is so much sugar hidden in our diets today, often in the form of high fructose corn syrup (or HFCS, on labels). Sugar is added to most processed foods, including crackers, cereals, canned fruit, some meats, soups, sauces, and salad dressings. Although nutrition labels don't offer a daily recommended percentage, steer clear of products that contain more than 10 grams of added sugar per serving. It's important to remember that low-fat dairy and fruits contain natural sugars—you may have heard of lactose and fructose—that are encouraged as part of a healthy lifestyle.

Know Your Label Lingo

Labels on food packages are advertising opportunities, and food manufacturers often make products sound healthier than they really are to get you to buy them. Here are some popular nutritional claims on food packaging and what you need to know about them.

Fat-Free, Sodium-Free, Sugar-Free, Trans Fat–Free. These words sound good, but any of these terms followed by the word "free" is misleading because the FDA allows less than 0.5 gram of these nutrients per serving. Last time I checked, 0.5 is not zero! If you eat more than a recommended serving, in no time you could be ingesting multiple grams of an unhealthy ingredient.

Made with Real Fruit. Sounds healthy, right? Well, most foods that bear this label contain sugar, high fructose corn syrup, and food dyes. Food manufacturers can use this term so long as they include the word "flavoring" among the ingredients. There have even been several lawsuits over deceptive advertising. So don't be fooled—when possible, eat real fruit instead.

100% Natural or All Natural. Unfortunately, the word *natural* on a food label is absolutely meaningless, even when the label says *100% natural* or *all natural*. The FDA has no regulatory oversight of the word *natural*. And by no means does it mean organic or healthy. To tell if something is natural, read the label: Do you recognize any of the words? Would most of the items come out of Granny's garden? If yes, then it's probably all natural and all right to eat!

Organic. *Organic* is a label regulated by the FDA and assigned to foods that are produced without certain types of pesticides or chemical fertilizers and that do not contain genetically modified organisms (GMOs). Organic food production also supports farming methods that are environmentally sound.

It is important to realize that just because a product is labeled organic does not mean it is low fat or even healthy. It just means it was produced in a more environmentally friendly way. Organic sugar is still sugar, and organic processed foods can still cause weight gain.

In terms of nutritional quality, at this time there is no conclusive evidence that organic produce is superior to conventional produce. Do not be afraid of fruits or vegetables that are not produced organically. The benefits of eating fruits and vegetables in whatever form suits your family and budget far outweigh any risk linked to chemical exposure. To reduce pesticide residue, which some studies have linked to weight gain, wash all fruits and vegetables well under running water before eating, cutting, or cooking them. This food safety practice should be done whether produce is organic, conventional, or picked out of your own backyard.

Don't allow marketers to take advantage of your decision to become healthier. Remember, the truth always lies in the ingredients list!

Make Fiber Your Friend

Fiber, which is mainly what plants are made of, helps your body digest food, keeps you full and satisfied, and helps you absorb nutrients. It can also help lower your risk for diabetes and heart disease. Look for the word on the nutritional labels of breads and cereals in particular. Whole grains contain more fiber and protein than other grains, and they are less processed. Consider adding foods high in fiber—containing 5 grams or more per serving—to your diet, and get at least 25 grams of fiber per day. Great foods that offer 5 grams or more per serving include broccoli, bran flakes, pears with the skin on, raspberries, cooked split peas, lima beans, whole wheat spaghetti, and even turnip greens!

Feed Your Family Well for Less Than $150 a Week

A lot of folks assume that healthier foods are more expensive. They certainly can be, if you're the type of person who wants to splurge on wild salmon and organic kale ... but for most folks, healthy doesn't have to mean costly. In fact, according to a new study from the Harvard School of Public Health, it costs just $1.50 per person per day to eat more whole foods than processed foods. I know that's not nothing, but if you look at the bigger picture, you'll save much more than that on long-term health-care costs when you eat better. (Honestly? If you quit the habit of eating junk like Cheetos and honey buns, you'll have money to buy more wholesome foods!)

There are three ways to accomplish this: Plan, plan, and plan! Am I repeating myself? Good! This way you won't forget. Before you go to the supermarket, plan your meals for a week. The meal guide on page 157 will help you, but here are some more strategies to keep in mind when planning.

Tips for Healthy and Less Expensive Meals

- Check to see what foods you already have and make a list of only what you need.
- Look for discounts. We all know about coupons; check for deals in the newspaper and those free fliers that fill up your mailbox. Ask for a loyalty card. You can save a lot if you shop in the same store often. Generally, the most expensive food items on a shopping list are meat and seafood.
- Compare different brands and different sizes of the same brand. No need to supersize an item you will only use for one recipe.
- Sometimes, however, it is cheaper to buy in bulk. Family packs of chicken, steak, or fish and larger bags of potatoes and frozen vegetables are often the better deal.

Because they are meal staples, you're likely to use them before they spoil.

- Go back to the basics. Pre-prepared foods like instant grits, quick 1-minute oatmeal, and frozen dinners cost you more than if you were to make them from scratch. Take a little more time preparing meals and save big-time on cost.
- Cook once and eat all week. Prepare a large batch on Sunday, and freeze portions of it in individual containers. This can replace take-out meals.
- Use your leftovers. For instance, a roast chicken can become chicken tacos; leftover beef and rice can have a second life when incorporated into a stir-fry. Remember: Throwing out food is throwing away money!

Bang for the Buck

Many of the cheapest foods we eat and drink contain empty calories—calories from bad fats or added sugars. Still, there are plenty of cheap foods that are perfectly healthy; you just need to know what they are.

That's why the Shape Up Sisters recipe suggestions, which are located in the next chapter and in the Recipes section at the back of this book, factor in both nutrition and cost and are designed around items that give you the most nutritional value for your money. The recipes—designed for real people who live on a budget and work all day—are all easy to make, using ingredients that can be found in most grocery stores. To get you started, here's an honor roll of the best foods for the money.

Sweet potatoes. Baked, mashed, sliced and roasted, or added to stews, they're full of fiber and vitamins, plus iron and calcium. To give you an idea, an average sweet potato contains 14 grams of fiber, more than *700 percent* of your daily vitamin A requirements, and 65 percent of your daily vitamin C!

Frozen greens, such as spinach, green beans, peas, and broccoli. Using these veggies is an easy way to add vitamins and fiber to your diet. These items are often on sale, and you can buy them in bulk for greater savings. Add these to soups, pastas, and chilies if you don't love them straight up.

Dried beans. Navy beans, pinto beans, black-eyed peas—these user-friendly legumes can be cooked easily on their own (as any Southerner knows!) or added to other dishes. They're about 10 cents per serving, and a small bag can feed an entire family. Prepare them in large batches and freeze them for quick reheat and eat opportunities.

Oats. They can be made into oatmeal for breakfast or added to cookies and other desserts to make them healthier. Oats cost 13 cents per serving and are packed with fiber and protein. Regular oats tend to be cheaper than instant.

Brown rice. Brown and white rice come from the same grain, but white rice has shed its nutritionally rich bran and germ layers. Brown rice is higher than white in fiber, B vitamins, and other nutrients like the mineral magnesium, which helps with a lot of your body's functions, such as maintaining your blood pressure. You can replace pasta and potato side dishes with brown rice recipes; one pot made on a Sunday will last you half the week (and you can recycle your daily leftovers in a healthy stir-fry!). Buy in bulk to save.

Chicken legs and thighs. The cheapest part of the chicken is also the most flavorful. It has more fat than chicken breast, though, so be sure to remove the skin before cooking.

Catfish and tilapia. Lean, full of protein, cheap, and widely available, these fish can be prepared in many ways.

Chuck. Red meat should be used sparingly, but when you need beef, pound for pound, chuck is the best value. It's not the leanest cut, so save it for use in lasagnas and other dishes where meat isn't the center.

This should help you get started on planning your meals.

Stay on Track When Dining Out

No, I don't expect that you'll always be staying at home to eat. Luckily, eating healthfully at restaurant chains is easier than it used to be, but you still have to watch portions and know how to order.

Often, healthy options are labeled with icons, such as a heart, or relegated to "healthy" or "lite" menu selections. At many national chain restaurants, nutritional values can be found on the menu or online. If no values are provided, you can ask your server if this information is available. Adults should limit a meal to 500 calories and children should stay under 350 calories.

When you order, get it *your* way. Not only are you paying for the meal, you have to wear the excess calories home. Your best bets are fish, chicken, and vegetarian options. Order them steamed, grilled, or broiled instead of fried or sautéed. Start your meal with a veggie-packed salad to help control hunger. Keep in mind that every tablespoon of mayonnaise, salad dressing, butter, and oil contains around 100 calories, so ask for them on the side so you can dip rather than drip in them.

What about when dining out is more than an excuse not to cook dinner, like a romantic date? An anniversary? A birthday celebration? Listen, my attitude is that a splurge every once in a while is good for the soul, and it actually helps you stay on track since you don't completely deprive yourself of the most indulgent foods and crave them constantly. So when you're being treated to a nice meal, your biggest worry should be which fork to use! But if you're really focused on getting your eating under control and want to stay on track, keep the following in mind:

- Moderation is the key to eating what you want. Order à la carte when available, since portions are generally smaller. Or order an appetizer for your main dish.
- Take a slice of bread, then give the basket back to the server. Choose an appetizer or dessert (not both), and toast with wine or light beer.
- Always drink plenty of water, and never skip meals leading up to dinner.

Most of all, remember that whether it's in the grocery store or at a restaurant, the choices are always *yours* to make.

The Myth of the Low Cost of Fast Food

People tend to believe that eating at fast-food restaurants is cheaper than buying groceries and cooking at home. But that's a big misconception. Though the dollar menu may *seem* like a bargain, it's never as inexpensive as buying the ingredients and making your own value meal at home. A 2010 study in the journal *Family Medicine* compared the cost of "convenience food" to whole foods and concluded that, "on a per-calorie basis, a convenience (fast-food) diet is more expensive than a diet derived from generic brand or frozen foods." Besides, there are the hidden costs that will become evident later—the cost to your health and your waistline.

But it doesn't take a whole team of researchers to do the math. See the chart on the next page for a side-by-side comparison.*

Fast Food	Homemade
McDonald's cheeseburger and french fries for family of four Cost: approximately $10	Homemade cheeseburgers and french fries for family of four Cost: approximately $4
KFC fried chicken and mashed potatoes for family of four Cost: approximately $20	Homemade oven-fried chicken and mashed potatoes for family of four Cost: approximately $8
Taco Bell tacos and chips and salsa for family of four Cost: approximately $12	Homemade tacos and chips and salsa for family of four Cost: approximately $4
Popeye's popcorn shrimp, beans and rice, and biscuits for family of four Cost: approximately $20	Homemade popcorn shrimp, beans and rice, and biscuits for family of four Cost: approximately $17

*Based on an average of estimates drawn from various regional supermarkets and fast food chains.

Part 3
The Shape Up Sisters Plan

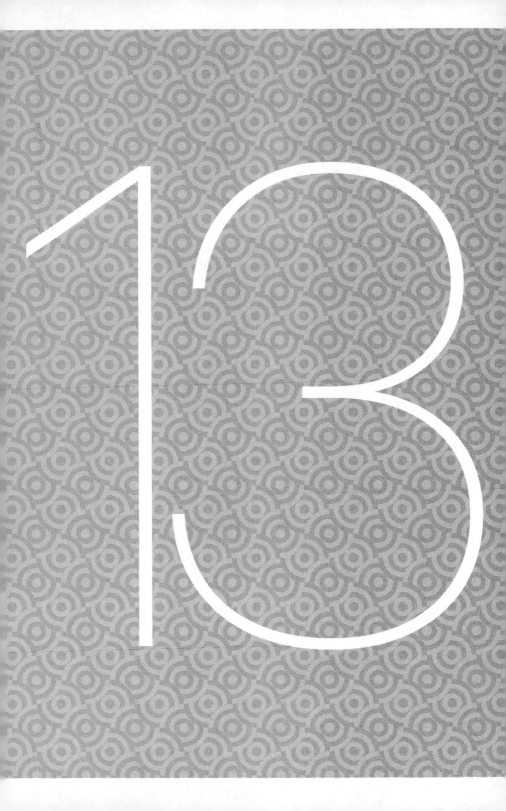

Eat Up!

The Food Plan

IN THE PREVIOUS SECTION OF THE BOOK, YOU
learned some strategies for being better prepared so that
you can feed yourself and your family well. You now
know how to shop smarter at the supermarket and how to
read label lingo so that you can make healthier decisions for
you and your family.

A nutritious, well-balanced eating plan is key to improving overall health. But where do you start? Does it mean you'll
be eating all brown rice and broccoli from now on? Absolutely
not! You can still eat nearly all of the foods you love. You just
need to be sure to balance your plate so you're not eating too
much of the foods that don't do you any favors and more of
the foods that will fuel you to have more energy and to lose
weight. (You'll also need to cook them in ways that don't leave
them drenched in butter and oil—more on that in a minute.)

I want to be clear about one thing: This isn't some gim-
micky diet. You've tried so many of those, and nothing has

worked in the long term. You equate *diet* with *starving*. And when you're out-of-your-mind hungry from deprivation, you give in to cravings and mindless snacking. This cycle of imbalanced dietary choices is leaving you overweight, under-nourished, and exhausted.

It is also keeping you broke. The price of a full-size bag of Doritos is $4 and a Big Gulp is about $1.39—just a snack for some people. For less than that, you can get a roast chicken at Costco.

I developed the following Shape Up Sisters Plate with the guidance of Rebecca Turner, a registered dietitian and board certified specialist in sports dietetics with the Academy of Nutrition and Dietetics in Jackson, Mississippi. What we're laying out here is a nutritious approach to eating that's based on the current USDA recommendations and will serve you for a lifetime. Your whole family can eat this way. If you eat in a balanced and mindful fashion, controlling your portions and eating more of the good stuff and less of the bad stuff, first you will see that you stop gaining weight. And soon enough, the weight will start to come off.

Tell a Good Calorie from a Bad Calorie

You might be wondering why you get hungry soon after you eat. It may surprise you to learn that stuffing food into an empty stomach doesn't slow your hunger drive, at least not for any substantial amount of time. The efficient and ongoing digestion and absorption of nutrients from food does. Nutrients such as protein, carbohydrates, and fat, plus vitamins and minerals (more on all these in a minute) tell the brain that you are giving the body what it needs to survive. Otherwise, the brain is just going to cue the release of chemicals that tell you to eat more and more.

You've heard of a calorie: It just refers to the amount of energy a food will produce in the body. We need calories to survive! But a calorie can come with a lot of good nutrients, or a calorie can come with very few. Those calories that don't pack a lot of nutrients are called *empty calories*. These are typically high in added sugar and saturated or solid fats (the type that stay solid at room temperature, like butter, lard, shortening, and beef fat). Most Americans eat way too many of them—I'm talking cakes, cookies, soda, ice cream, pizza, and yes, fried chicken. When you load up on empty calories, your energy spikes and then drops and you're hungry again in no time. How's that so? Here's the bare-bones explanation of how digestion works.

When you eat food, your stomach breaks it down into *macronutrients*—proteins, fats, and carbohydrates. Next, the food enters your small intestine and is broken down even more, into vitamins and minerals. Then, the small intestine absorbs the nutrients into the bloodstream. From the bloodstream, they are sent to your liver, where they will be stored or sent to other parts of the body for use. What's left is sent to your large intestine, where any remaining water gets absorbed before the food is compounded into solid waste to be expelled from the body.

Meanwhile, the nutrients that passed through the small intestine and into the bloodstream are busy nourishing your body. When absorption is finally accomplished, blood sugar levels drop and send a signal to your brain. The brain triggers the red alert that food is needed. It is blood sugar dropping, not an empty stomach, that signals hunger. When you stabilize your blood sugar with nutrients, you stave off hunger.

What are some examples of nutrient-rich, good calories? Fruits and vegetables, whole wheat bread, baked chicken breast (without skin), 95 percent extra lean ground beef, unsweetened cereal, and low-fat or skim milk.

The more nutrients in a food, the more nutrition that is

available to be delivered throughout the body. So you can stay full and satisfied on fewer calories. Sure, you can have those empty calories once in a while; once again, the key is balance.

Know Your Food Groups

It seems to me sometimes that every woman knows how to diet but not how to actually eat. How should you fill your plate every day? What we're giving you here are the building blocks for a healthy diet. For the Shape Up Sisters Plate, we're simply adopting the USDA's MyPlate plan, because it is so easy to follow using a familiar icon that you have in front of you virtually every time you eat. (For a look at the plate icon, see page 144.) Print out the icon from **choosemyplate.gov** and tape it to your fridge or pantry. Look at it regularly until you commit it to memory!

Here are the food groups that you need to know. We will tell you how they all should come together on your plate in a minute.

Protein

Protein is the only nutrient capable of repairing and creating muscle mass. It's simple: If you don't eat quality protein, you won't build quality muscle. You need lean muscle because it's the furnace where calories are burned up and energy is stored—even when you are not doing anything but sitting on the couch. Without enough muscle, weight loss or maintenance is impossible and exhaustion is inevitable. Studies show that we lose up to 1 percent of muscle mass each year, starting in our thirties! Good nutrition and exercise can reverse this decline. Protein can also help curb hunger because it takes longer to digest than some of those empty-calorie foods I mentioned.

You should be eating a variety of foods rich in protein every day. High-protein foods include lean cuts of meat (beef, pork, veal, and lamb), poultry (chicken or turkey), seafood (fish and shrimp), eggs, low-fat dairy (milk, yogurt, and cheese), nuts and seeds, beans, and soy (tofu).

So how much protein should you eat? The amount depends on age, gender, and activity level. The Centers for Disease Control suggests that on average women require 46 grams a day and men, 56 grams a day. But you don't need to constantly tally it all up—that can make your head hurt, and besides, most Americans get more than enough protein for their basic needs. If you just focus on eating healthy proteins, such as those listed below, you'll find it's very easy to hit those levels by eating foods you love.

1 chicken breast = 30 grams
1 egg = 6 grams
1 ground beef patty (4 ounces) = 28 grams
1 can (6 ounces) of tuna = 40 grams
½ cup of cooked beans = about 8 grams (black, pinto, lentils)

Protein should take up one-quarter of your plate. From now on, ask yourself, Where is my protein? when planning a menu, fixing a plate, or ordering at a restaurant.

Grains

Grains are carbohydrates—everyone's favorite type of food. Foods made from wheat, rice, oats, cornmeal, or barley are all grains (and therefore carbohydrates). Although carbs have gotten a bad rap in the last decade, the truth is that nobody can afford to skip them, since your body breaks them down into sugars to give you energy for your daily activities and exercise, plus they boost blood sugar levels and keep the brain working at full throttle.

However, there are good and not-so-great choices. I'm sure you know what I'm talking about.

Grains are divided into two types: whole grains and refined grains. Whole grains are closest to how grains are found in nature and contain the entire kernel, where most of the nutrition is located. That's why whole grains are typically brown. **Examples of whole grains include:**

Barley
Brown rice
Oatmeal
Popcorn
Whole wheat bread
Whole wheat cereal

Refined grains have been processed to remove that healthy outer hull and germ, which keeps products from spoiling but strips grain of most of its vitamins and fiber. That's why refined grains tend to be white or yellow. These include all the foods we love to indulge in. **Examples of refined grains include:**

Cornbread
Cornflakes
White bread
White flour pasta
White rice

Understanding how the body uses and stores carbohydrates can help you see why too much, particularly of the wrong kind, is not a good thing. The body breaks down carbohydrates—from both whole and refined grains—into sugars, which get absorbed into the bloodstream. Once there, the pancreas is signaled to release a surge of insulin. Think of insulin as your "sugar train": Its job is to go through the blood and pick up excess "sugar passengers." Over time, if the train never leaves the station or there are more passengers than available seats, you can develop type 2 diabetes.

The sugar that gets on the sugar train fuels the muscles and brain. However, if there is too much of it at any given time, or if your muscles are unable to burn through it through walking or some other activity or exercise, it will be stored as fat! Did a lightbulb go off? The extra dinner roll, the second helping of pie, and the mindless potato chip munching cause the trouble. Eating throughout the day in a balanced way, and not filling up on too many carbohydrates at once, allows your energy to be used through daily activity or exercise.

One other key thing to know is that the thing that slows down the flood of sugar onto the sugar train and into the bloodstream is fiber—which is what that brown hull on whole grains is. (Fiber is also found in fruits and vegetables, beans, and nuts.) So the more you eat whole grain, high-fiber carbohydrates, the happier your digestive tract will be on the inside and the leaner you'll be on the outside!

Grains should take up one-quarter of your plate. From now on when you're planning a meal, ask, "Where is my grain?"

Vegetables

Three words: Eat 'em up!

Vegetables are full of vitamins, minerals, fiber, and phytochemicals (disease fighters), and they offer relatively few calories. Countless studies have shown that a diet rich in a variety of vegetables can protect against diabetes, obesity, and certain kinds of cancer.

There are many types of vegetables. The USDA divides them into five categories.

Dark green vegetables: These include dark leafy greens (like collards and kale), broccoli, Brussels sprouts, green beans, lettuce, and spinach. This is the category that tends to get the most groans, but the best part is that they can be made to be delicious, and you don't need any portion control!

Red and orange vegetables: Squash, carrots, sweet potatoes, tomatoes, and red peppers are in this group. Like dark green vegetables, these are highly nutritious (their bright color gives them different disease-fighting properties than greens), and you can eat as much of them as you want.

Starchy vegetables: Corn, green peas, and potatoes make up most of this category. They're called "starchy" because they contain less fiber per serving than nonstarchy vegetables. That doesn't mean they're bad— just don't fill up every time on only starchy vegetables or you'll be missing the amazing weight-control and disease-fighting powers of the other types of vegetables.

Beans and peas: Foods like black beans, kidney beans, pinto beans, white beans, black-eyed peas, garbanzo beans, and lentils are different from other vegetables because they are especially high in protein—on a level with meat sources! So on one hand, you could consider these part of the protein foods group and use them as vegetarian alternatives to meat and poultry. On the other hand, they are on the vegetable list because their nutrient content—the phytochemicals and fiber—are comparable to those of vegetables. Don't get bogged down worrying about which group to put them in. They can count for either group toward filling out the MyPlate icon.

As I noted in the last chapter, fresh produce is great if you can get it, but you can also feel good about including any vegetables that are frozen or canned in water. They are all healthy. Bake, boil, microwave, grill, sauté, steam, or eat them raw; just make sure you eat them often.

Vegetables should cover a little more than one-quarter of your plate. From now on, ask yourself, "Where are my vegetables?"

Fruits

Like vegetables, fruits are rich in nutrients for disease prevention, relatively low in calories, and an important part of a weight-loss plan. Yes, fruit tastes sweet, but the sugar in fruit, called fructose, is bound up with a lot of fiber, which slows that rush of sugar to that sugar train so the pancreas isn't overwhelmed. Fiber also has a ton of health benefits, including helping to ward off cancer and diabetes. So don't be afraid of fruit just because some crazy diets in the past have told you to limit it! It's highly unlikely that you are going to eat a dozen apples or bananas in one sitting, so consider fruit to be on your free-to-eat list.

Try to get a range of fruits in your diet—everything from apples and pears to peaches and pineapple are fair game. In season—when they are cheaper and also taste better—melons and berries are great choices, too. But frozen fruit is a great runner-up, as is fruit canned in its own juice.

Fruit should take up a little less than one-quarter of your plate (a little less than vegetables because of its sugar). Fruit is a good way to get kids used to eating something healthy at dinner and is an excellent replacement snack when your sweet tooth just won't stop nagging you.

Dairy

Not to confuse you, but dairy contains both protein and carbohydrates. Yet on the USDA MyPlate it gets its own little category. Why? Because foods in this group—namely milk, cheese, and yogurt—contain nutrients that are really important to health, particularly bone health. These include calcium and vitamin D, which are particularly crucial for women and children. The amount you need depends on age and gender, but the USDA recommends that adults and kids older than 9 get 3 cups a day. (Children younger than 9 need a little less.)

People with lactose intolerance—which affects well over half of the general population and upwards of 75 percent of

African Americans, Latinos, and Asian Americans—should know that when it comes to milk, a few practical solutions can help: Drinking lactose-free milk, which comes in various fat levels and flavors, is real milk, just without the lactose. And you can try to gradually reintroduce milk into the diet by trying small amounts with food or by cooking with it. You can also substitute soy milk here if dairy is not your thing, since it is also rich in calcium and protein. Dairy choices should be low fat or fat free, because consuming high levels of saturated fats isn't good for heart health.

Of course, vegans will skip the dairy; just be sure to get extra protein through more plant-based, protein-rich foods like beans and soy, and calcium through dark leafy greens.

The Skinny on Fat

Before getting into how to put your plate together to create balanced meals, you need to understand a few things about dietary fat, as in the kind you eat. Butter, oil, margarine, lard—in the South, we all know about cooking with fat! But it's more complicated than that: During the 1980s there was a dieting trend that had us believing that simply eating fat made us fat. People went to great lengths to reduce and remove fat from their diets, and manufacturers did the same with their products. Often fat was replaced with sugar or salt to make foods, like cookies or soups, taste good. This shift did not solve our obesity or heart disease problems; in fact, it only made things worse. People thought that low-fat options were healthier, so they could be eaten in greater quantities.

Well, it turns out that dietary fat is necessary for sustaining life. Fat acts as a hunger suppressor, absorbs and transports certain vitamins to the body's cells, and protects vital organs. Did you know our brains are made up of 60 percent fat? To function in high gear, our brains need to maintain this level of fat. In fact, a lower amount can lead to neurological disorders.

But does that mean you need your deep fryer? Heck no! Put that thing away. Let's be reasonable here. Just like whole grains and fruits are good carbs and chicken breast is a better protein than ground beef, some fats are better than others. Portion control is essential here, too.

Fat that comes from animal sources—such as butter, bacon grease, and lard—is known as *saturated fat*. You can tell if something is a saturated fat because it will be white and solid when it is not heated. Saturated fat raises your body's HDL (or "bad") cholesterol. Too much of the bad type of cholesterol is harmful to your heart and circulatory system and can lead to heart disease and other health issues.

A better choice for a dietary fat source? Think of plants first. Avocados, olives, nuts, seeds, and oils from plants (such as olive oil or canola) contain *unsaturated fat*. This type of fat remains liquid at room temperature and does not contain any cholesterol. In fact, unsaturated fat is thought to *lower* HDL or "bad" cholesterol in the body.

Another type of fat has been in the news lately: *trans fats*. These are created through a process called hydrogenation, which makes the oil less likely to spoil. Manufacturers can keep foods on a shelf longer by using trans fats. But enough science has proven trans fats are a health risk, and now the United States is moving to join European countries like Denmark and Switzerland in banning them.

They are still in foods, however. To remove them from your diet, start by looking at the ingredients list on food labels. *Partially hydrogenated oil* is just another term for trans fat.

Now that you are aware of which dietary fats to choose and avoid, you are probably wondering how much fat is okay to eat.

Here's the answer: Use common sense! Fat is calorie dense, meaning that just a little gives you a lot of fuel. Skip the butter when you can and replace it with healthier oils, like olive oil. When you can't or don't want to pass on the butter, use half of what you usually use and aim to go down from there. When preparing food, save fried food, heavily sautéed food, bacon, lard, and cream sauces for very special occasions.

Putting It All on Your Shape Up Sisters Plate

Now that you know the major components of healthy eating, how do you put them together? As I noted, I am simply using the USDA's well-established MyPlate guidelines as a basis for demonstrating what a balanced and satisfying meal looks like. I want you to use this plan to make every meal healthy, convenient, and inexpensive. It's easy to understand, easy to remember, and the USDA.gov site has lots more information on how to make healthy choices.

We've gone over the what, the why, and the how, so let's review what your plate should look like when you're sitting down to a meal:

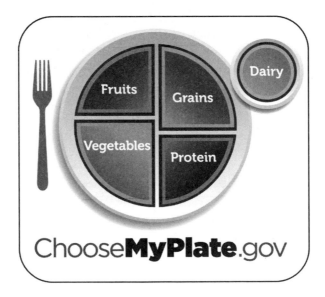

- One-half of your plate will be fruits and vegetables—with more veggies than fruit.
- One-quarter of your plate will be filled with protein foods.
- One-quarter of your plate will be filled with grains.
- On the plate or in a glass, low-fat dairy foods should be a part of each meal.

Now, as I mentioned, some foods have both protein and carbohydrates—like milk and beans and peas—but let's not get too complicated here. Memorizing the look of this plate will help you stay out of trouble and keep your meals the most nutritious they can be.

These practical, healthy, and tasty guidelines—which can be used every day, at every meal—will help you reach and maintain your ideal weight and reduce your risk of chronic disease. Don't forget, this program is not a diet but a tool to teach you how to eat. Our culture places too much emphasis on strict dieting and not enough on learning how to eat well.

Like I've said before, the first goal is to stop weight gain; then, as you become more comfortable and confident, you will see weight loss start to kick in. Incorporate these principles into your everyday eating habits and you won't feel that crazy hunger anymore, because your blood sugar will be more stable, and you won't feel like you're deprived, like on some silly diet that has you only drinking powdered shakes twice a day.

Success is not about perfection, but consistency. The key is not to control every circumstance, but to respond to it in a balanced way.

Preparing to Eat Up

For a Southerner, food is a way of life. Here in the South, all traditions and social events revolve around food. We meet to eat! Hours are spent around the kitchen table catching up and celebrating. Family recipes are time-honored traditions and become ingrained in our memories, and we all dream of our favorite dishes.

Most people believe that eating traditional Southern cuisine makes you fat, but it doesn't have to be that way. Here are a few tricks from dietitian Rebecca Turner to make over any recipe to complement a healthy eating lifestyle. (And remember: Although recipes can be made healthier, you still need to be mindful of portion control.)

- If a recipe calls for pasta, use half and add more vegetables.
- Add extra vegetables to any casserole, soup, or stew.
- Switch to low-fat milk, 2% cheese, light butter, or fat-free condensed soups.
- Switch to brown rice and 100% whole wheat noodles and bread crumbs.
- Leave sauces and dressings on the side for individual serving at the table.
- "Oven fry" or roast meat, fish, potatoes, and vegetables instead of deep frying.
- Replace half the ground meat in tacos, spaghetti, or casseroles with beans.
- Replace white potatoes with sweet potatoes—so much more nutritious!
- Replace ham bones and bacon with ¼ cup olive oil in a large pot to cook collards, mustard greens, and cabbage.
- Reduce 1 cup of sugar to ⅔ cup in baked goods, and add extra flavor by using vanilla, traditional baking spices, or fruit.
- Reduce fat in baked goods and add flavor by replacing some of the butter or oil recommendations with Greek yogurt, canned pumpkin puree, or applesauce. (Exactly how much depends on the recipe, but a good rule of thumb is to replace no more than half of the original fat.)

- Use spray butter or healthy oil spritzers (such as canola or grape-seed oil) to flavor food instead of tablespoons of butter, shortening, or corn oil; it will limit how much you use.

A Guide to Portion Size

Portion sizes have gotten out of control. But you already have on hand all you need to control portion sizes. Literally. It turns out that your own hand is the best tool for estimating portion size. Here's how.

- Make a fist—that's about 1 cup, the recommended portion size of grains per meal.
- The palm of your hand is a cooked serving of meat.
- The tip of your thumb equals 1 teaspoon (a serving of mayonnaise, for example).
- Cup your hand. This makes one serving of nuts.
- The length of your hand is the proper fish fillet portion.
- The length of your hand is also a good guide to measure white and sweet potatoes.

And consider these strategies for reining in the amount you and your family eat at meals and in between.

- Purchase single-serving snacks, or portion out snacks into bags or cups before eating.
- Leave serving dishes on the stove rather than putting them on the table, family-style. This will minimize the temptation for second helpings.
- Divide up dinner leftovers before putting them in the refrigerator for easy-to-grab lunches.
- Portions of casseroles, soups, stews, or spaghetti should equal 1 to 1½ cups.

A Note on Plate Size

Since we're talking about changing what's on your plate, you may also need to change your plate itself and downsize your dinnerware. The surface area of dinner plates has increased 36 percent since 1960, from an average of 9 inches to 12 inches today! Larger dinnerware has led to portion sizes that are far bigger than what we need. Instead, eat your main meals from salad plates.

Similarly, the Big Gulp mentality has changed how we drink at home. Drink sweetened beverages from 8-ounce glasses and stick to one glass per meal. Of course, if you're drinking water, which is a great choice for families—just put a pitcher on the table!—your glass can be as big as you like.

Better Kitchen Staples

If you stock your pantry, fridge, and freezer with healthier options, then you will always have something good on hand to eat and won't have to hop in the car for takeout (or be tempted by crackers, chips, and cookies calling your name). Cut back on processed foods—cookies, crackers, chips, yes, all of these favorite snacks!—to reduce your dietary intake of sugar, salt, bad fats, and refined grains, all of which are an express ticket to obesity, diabetes, and other chronic health problems. Buy healthy options in quantities you will eat before they go bad.

PROTEINS

Canned meat in water: Tuna, salmon, sardines, chicken
Chicken and turkey legs: When on special, buy and freeze
Eggs: Large cartons save money and last
Lean (95%) ground meat (beef, turkey): When on special, buy and freeze
Low-fat Greek yogurt:
Individual cartons (can last 2 weeks)
Low-fat cottage cheese: Individual cartons (can last 2 weeks)
Low-fat string cheese: Large bag (can last 2 to 3 weeks)

Natural nut butter: Should contain only peanuts (or almonds or cashews) and salt

Skinless chicken or turkey breast: When on special, buy and freeze

Unsalted nuts and seeds: Almonds, walnuts, pecans, sunflower seeds, pumpkin seeds

Canned beans: black beans, chickpeas, kidney beans, lentils

HEALTHY GRAINS

Whole grain pasta: Look for 5 grams of fiber per serving

Whole grains: Barley, brown rice, old-fashioned oatmeal (not instant), whole cornmeal

Whole wheat bread: Look for breads without high fructose corn syrup

Whole wheat wraps and tortillas: Look for 5 grams of fiber per serving

VEGETABLES AND FRUIT

Favorite green and red or orange vegetables:
- Canned should be no or low sodium
- Fresh should only be purchased a week's worth at a time to avoid spoilage
- Frozen (broccoli, spinach, Brussels sprouts, green beans, stir-fry mix) are so easy to quickly zap in the microwave

Favorite starchy vegetables: frozen or canned (corn, peas, butter beans)

Favorite fruit:
- As with fresh vegetables, buy only what you can eat in a week
- Canned should be 100% juice and not in syrup or "cocktail" mixtures
- Dried unsweetened fruits, like raisins, prunes, cranberries
- Frozen unsweetened fruit or fruit mix is a great option and easy to just pop into a blender for smoothies

HEART-HEALTHY FATS

Extra-virgin olive oil

Extra-virgin olive oil spray

Light butter: Ingredients should include only milk, cream, and salt

Light dressings: Avoid partially hydrogenated oils (trans fats) and high fructose corn syrup

Light mayonnaise

OTHER

Balsamic vinegar

Dried spices for extra flavor

Ground pepper

Salsa

Stone-ground mustard

Menu Planning 101

A coach never takes the field without a game plan, so don't start the week without a menu plan. You can't eat what's not there. When you have healthy options in the house, you omit the give-in guilt and comfort food–filled dinnertime. Not to mention, you save time and money. But menu planning can be time-consuming and tedious. Give it some time; it will become a habit, I promise.

Use these tips to menu plan for success.

- Sketch out an ideal healthy meal.
- Pick a menu planning day and block off time in your schedule.
- Don't feel you have to be wildly creative and serve up something original every single day. Do what's realistic and won't stress you out. If you have a few go-to healthy recipes that everyone likes, rely on them and expand your recipes gradually.
- Make extra so you can use the leftovers the next day (or freeze the extra).
- Pencil in dining out so it's not a frequent fallback plan.

Better Plate Menus

Here are some menu ideas from Rebecca Turner that balance out the different food groups we've been over. Most lunches and dinners incorporate protein, whole grains, vegetables and/or fruits, and a dairy option. Breakfasts and snacks are simpler and typically contain a protein and whole grain, and sometimes a fruit or vegetable.

The possible combinations are endless, so use these as inspiration to figure out how to modify your favorite recipes to hit all the food groups. And see page 208 for delicious ideas for Southern recipe makeovers!

BREAKFAST

- 2 scrambled eggs, 1 whole wheat English muffin, apple butter spread, 1 cup milk
- 1 ounce turkey sausage, 1 cup grits, ½ teaspoon butter, 1 medium orange
- 2 slices whole wheat toast, 1 tablespoon natural peanut butter, 1 medium banana
- 1 cup low-fat yogurt, ½ cup light granola, 1 cup cubed fruit
- ½ cup 2% cottage cheese, 1 medium whole grain muffin, 1 cup sliced peaches (fresh or canned in water)
- 2 slices turkey bacon, 2 slices whole wheat toast, 2 or 3 slices tomato
- 1 cup low-fat milk, 1 serving whole grain cereal, ½ cup 100% orange juice
- 4 egg whites or scrambled tofu, 1 whole wheat pita pocket, ¼ avocado
- 6 ounces Greek yogurt, 2 sliced kiwis, ¼ cup dark chocolate nibs
- 1 cup oatmeal, 1 cup milk, 1 tablespoon natural peanut or other nut butter
- 1 cup cooked grits, ½ cup Cheddar cheese, 1 cup mixed berries

LUNCH

Endless salad combinations: 3 to 4 ounces lean meat or other protein (fish, poultry, low-fat cheese, tofu), 1 serving whole grain crackers, mixed salad greens, 1 tablespoon light dressing, 1 medium fruit

Endless sandwich combinations: 3 to 4 ounces lean meat or other protein (fish, poultry, low-fat cheese, tofu), 2 slices whole wheat bread, lettuce, tomatoes, onion, 1 tablespoon light mayonnaise, 1 low-fat yogurt

Endless pita or wrap combinations: 3 to 4 ounces lean meat or other protein (fish, poultry, low-fat cheese, tofu), whole wheat pita pocket or 6-inch whole wheat wrap, lettuce, tomatoes, onion, 1 tablespoon light mayonnaise

Endless soup and salad combinations: 1½ cups of noncream-based soups, side salad, 1 tablespoon light dressing, 1 cup cubed fruit

Veggie burger: 1 veggie burger patty, 1 whole wheat hamburger bun, spinach, red onion, tomato, ¼ cup sliced avocado, 1 tablespoon light Dijon mustard, 1 medium pear

Vegetarian wrap: Sautéed tofu or ½ cup beans, 1 whole wheat wrap, endless nonstarchy vegetables, 1 ounce Cheddar cheese, ½ cup unsweetened applesauce

Breakfast for lunch—omelet: 4 egg whites, 2 slices whole wheat toast, assorted chopped vegetables, ¼ cup part-skim mozzarella cheese

PB&J: 1 tablespoon peanut butter or other nut butter, 2 slices whole wheat bread, 1 tablespoon no-sugar-added jelly

DINNER

Grilled meat with rice: 1 portion grilled seafood or lean meat, ½ cup brown rice, vegetable medley

Healthy stir-fry: Sautéed shrimp, beef, or chicken and ½ cup each mushrooms, snap peas, carrot matchsticks, and onions sautéed in 1 tablespoon extra-virgin olive oil, served over ½ cup quinoa or brown rice

Baked salmon: 1 portion baked salmon (with 1 teaspoon butter), 1 medium baked sweet potato (with 1 teaspoon butter), roasted asparagus

Healthy cheeseburger: Ground 95%+ lean beef patty, 1 whole wheat bun, lettuce, tomato, onion, side salad with vegetables, 1 ounce low-fat Swiss cheese, 1 tablespoon light dressing, mustard

Veggie spaghetti: Take your favorite spaghetti recipe and substitute beans for meat and whole wheat spaghetti for regular pasta

Steak and potatoes: 3 to 4 ounces sirloin steak, 1 medium baked potato, 1 cup steamed broccoli, 1 teaspoon butter, 1 tablespoon light sour cream

Healthy tacos: Lean ground turkey (cooked in taco seasoning), 2 corn taco shells, lettuce, tomato, onions, ¼ cup shredded cheese, 1 tablespoon light sour cream, salsa

Healthy Mexican salad: 1 portion chicken, beef, or shrimp, ½ cup black beans, chopped tomatoes and cucumbers, 2 cups lettuce of choice, ¼ cup sliced avocado, 1 tablespoon sour cream, salsa

Healthy fajitas: 1 portion chicken, beef, or shrimp, 2 soft tortillas, chopped tomatoes and cucumbers, 2 cups lettuce of choice, ¼ cup guacamole, 1 tablespoon sour cream, salsa

Healthy fish fillets: Baked fish fillets, baked sweet potato fries, large side salad, 1 tablespoon light dressing

Healthy fried chicken: Oven-baked fried chicken, oven-roasted plum tomatoes, sliced cornbread, ¼ cup pesto

SNACKS

- ¼ cup almonds and 1 medium apple
- ½ cup hummus and unlimited raw veggies
- 1 cheese stick and air-popped popcorn
- 1 cup low-fat Greek yogurt and 1 medium banana
- ½ cup 2% cottage cheese and 1 cup sliced peaches (fresh or canned in water)
- ½ cup black bean dip and 1 serving baked chips
- ½ cup dark chocolate nibs and ¼ cup dried fruit
- 1 tablespoon natural peanut butter and 2 rice cakes
- ¼ cup walnuts and 1 small box raisins
- 1 cup natural salsa and 1 serving baked chips

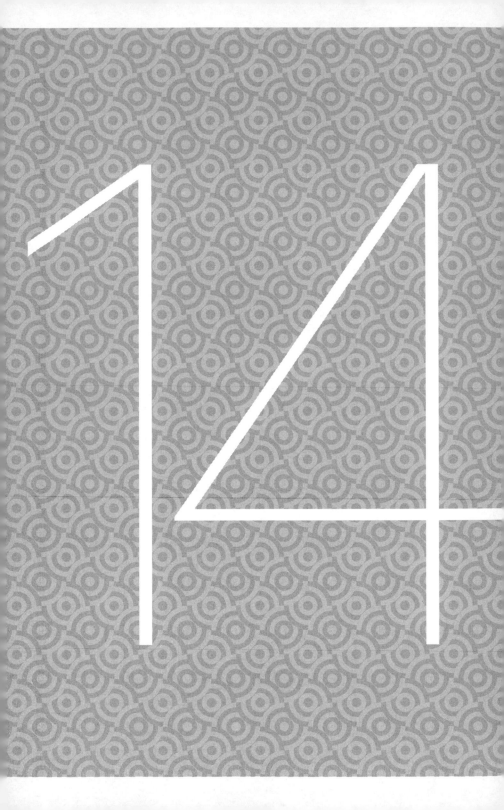

Shape Up!

The Fitness Plan

NOW THAT YOU HAVE A PLAN FOR EXERCISING your brain with positive thinking and nourishing your body with nutritious food, here's a plan for shaping up your body. All three work together to improve your health and quality of life.

Starting an exercise program can be scary. I've heard fear in the voices of many women who come to my gym after getting troubling diagnoses from their doctors. Most have had a negative experience with exercise in the past or just see it as another form of stress in their lives. The question to ask yourself is, if you are too broken down and sick, and can't meet the needs of those counting on you, who will?

Take Ebony. When she was barely 20, she moved with her mother to Vicksburg after her mother was injured at work and needed care. Caretaking can be incredibly demanding, and Ebony soon noticed that she had put on weight and felt changes in her self-esteem.

"I went to the doctor for my annual exam and the medical assistant asked me, 'How much do you weigh?' I proudly answered, '200 pounds!' She looked at me as though I was crazy and told me to step on the scale. I did, and it read 310. I felt my heart drop to the floor. I was hurt and disappointed in myself. I could not understand how I had gained so much weight. Following the appointment, I asked my mother how much she thought I weighed and she answered, 'Around 220 or 240.' I laughed, but on the inside I was crying. Once we arrived home, I told her that we had to talk. I told her that I weighed 310 pounds and that I had to lose weight or I was going to die. My poor eating habits and lack of physical activity were what would kill me.

"We both made the decision to change our eating habits, but I knew that we also had to start some form of physical activity. I went to Shape Up Sisters and purchased a membership. My mother insisted that she was too old to exercise, no matter how much I tried to convince her otherwise. After weeks of her sitting in the gym watching me exercise, noticing the results and the staff members' encouragement, my mother joined the gym. We began our weight-loss journey together. We also decided to become vegetarians and today our diets consist of vegetables, plenty of fruit, fish and water.... Along this journey, we have run into many obstacles, especially finances and staying on the right path. But over the past 6 months, I have lost 50 pounds and counting. My mother has lost 30 pounds. No, the journey isn't over. It has just begun."

I can't stress it enough: Exercise will change you on the inside and outside and can add years to your life. Good health is yours for the asking, but you have to believe that change is possible and obey the simple goals you set for yourself.

If you are a beginner—that is, if you have been exercising for less than 6 months, or if you have been exercising inconsistently—there are a few things you should consider first.

1. Do you have any health or medical conditions that will prevent you from exercising? Being physically active is safe for most people, but you may need to check with your doctor before starting an exercise program.

2. Where will you exercise? At the gym, your home, at work, in a park?

3. What time of day will you be able to exercise? Before work, after work, at lunch? You'll need to find a way to budget the time and stick to it.

4. Do you need social support? Consider whether you could use the help of a friend, group fitness environment, personal trainer, or community programs.

5. Are you truly ready to exercise? If you believe you can do it and truly commit, success will be so much easier.

These questions will help you start off on the right foot. Laziness is a self-defeating behavior, so you have to be tough on yourself and avoid making excuses. Visualizing yourself doing what you most want to do helps. And don't forget to sign the Shape Up Sisters contract and hang it on your fridge or someplace prominent in your house so when you start to backslide, your goal will be staring you in the face!

The goal of this chapter is to help you improve your health by meeting the surgeon general's physical activity guidelines, which are a minimum of 30 minutes of moderate-intensity aerobic activity (like brisk walking) five times a week and strength training that works all major muscle groups (legs, hips, back, abdomen, chest, shoulders, and arms) at least twice a week. If you are meeting those requirements, then you are ready to move up to even greater health benefits. The Shape Up workout can show you how to do both.

In addition, the workout is designed to promote what's known as functional exercise. By doing functional fitness, you will reinforce the types of movements you do in everyday life:

climbing stairs, carrying your children, reaching for and picking up objects, vacuuming, pushing a heavy grocery cart from one end of a parking lot to another, playing a sport, or working in the garden. When you don't work out, your ability to do simple daily tasks decreases and your risk of injury goes up.

The workout has two parts: a schedule to get you walking and a workout to do at home. If you do all the exercises, which include a combination of cardio, strength, balance, coordination, and flexibility, you'll reduce your risk of developing chronic illnesses, such as heart disease, diabetes, and cancer. I've heard it said that if exercise could be packaged in a pill, it would be the most widely prescribed medication in the world!

This workout will also help you make a long-term commitment to fitness. Starting small and then building on it really does bring results. So let's get started!

Let's Go Walking

Walking is the number one exercise in the world. It is what our bodies were designed to do—even more so than running. All you need is a pair of good walking shoes and the desire to move. Walking can be done at any time—on your own or with others. There are huge health and emotional benefits to being outdoors and connecting with nature, family, and friends. Haven't seen your mom in a while? Invite her for a walk. Haven't been active in as long as you can remember? Start by just walking leisurely to your mailbox and back five times. Swing your arms and breathe. A 10-minute walk can boost your mood quickly, and the aftereffects can last throughout the day.

When you are comfortable, use the table below to get started on the Shape Up 4-week walking plan. By the end of Week 4, your walking time will equal 30 minutes, which meets the surgeon general's guidelines.

Beginner Walking Routine

Week	Warmup (Walk Easy)	Walk Fast	Cooldown (Walk Easy)
1	5 minutes	5 minutes	5 minutes
2	5 minutes	7 minutes	5 minutes
3	5 minutes	10 minutes	5 minutes
4	5 minutes	20 minutes	5 minutes

While walking, hold your head up and stand tall, trying not to lean forward. Look straight ahead, swing your arms with a slight bend in your elbows, and tuck in your tummy. Repeat this affirmation during your walk: "My health is my wealth."

If you are already walking and want to kick it up a notch, you can move from moderate to vigorous intensity by jogging. Or mix it up by walking some, then jogging some (see the "Beginner Walk/Run Routine" below). If you are pressed for time, a little-known rule of thumb is that 1 minute of vigorous-intensity activity is about the same as 2 minutes of moderate-intensity activity. So, if you walk for 15 minutes and jog for 15 minutes, that is equal to 45 minutes of exercise.

Beginner Walk/Run Routine

Week	Warmup (Walk Easy)	Walk Fast	Jog Easy	Walk Fast	Cooldown (Walk Easy)
1	5 minutes	10 minutes	1 minute	5 minutes	5 minutes
2	5 minutes	10 minutes	2 minutes	5 minutes	5 minutes
3	5 minutes	10 minutes	4 minutes	5 minutes	5 minutes
4	5 minutes	20 minutes	10 minutes	10 minutes	5 minutes

A pedometer is a great motivating tool to help you meet the physical activity guidelines. Aim for 10,000 steps a day, which is equal to 5 miles. Walk laps at the mall, at the grocery store, at a museum or park, or even around your kitchen and living room! It's fun to find ways to push your daily step count.

If you want to branch out beyond walking—to swimming, biking, dancing, jumping rope—by all means, do it! As you know from Chapter 11, variety is the key to fighting boredom and also to challenging your body in ways that will bring faster gains. There are so many ways to get your 30 minutes of moderate-intensity aerobic activity a day. Let's review some terms so you can find a routine that works best for you.

Aerobic activity or *"cardio"* gets you breathing harder and your heart beating faster. All types of activities count, so long as you do them at a moderate or vigorous intensity for at least *10 minutes* at a time.

Moderate-intensity aerobic activity does *not* mean shopping, cooking, doing laundry, or sitting on a lawnmower; your body just isn't working hard enough during these activities to get your heart rate up. During a moderate-intensity activity, you should be able to talk, but not sing the words to your favorite song.

Vigorous-intensity aerobic activity means you're breathing hard and fast and your heart rate has gone up quite a bit. If you are at this level, you shouldn't be able to say more than a few words without pausing for a breath. Examples of vigorous activities are running, swimming laps, and riding a bike up a hill.

Remember, if you haven't been active lately, increase your activity level slowly. You need to feel comfortable doing moderate-intensity activities before you move on to more vigorous ones. Keep in mind that your workout should be about doing physical activity that feels right for you.

Home Circuit

A lot of gyms, including my own, offer what's called a circuit workout. It is a great option because it combines cardio training with strength training. This allows you to get more done in less time. Circuit training is great for all fitness levels and is especially used for weight loss programs. Best of all, you don't need a gym to do it! You just need your own body weight, a space to move in, and a few household objects. Even more important, creativity and a good sense of humor can lead to fun and fulfilling workouts.

If you would like to join a gym but are afraid you won't fit in or can't keep up, then this workout will help you gain the confidence to join one.

The fitness goal for this workout is to exercise all of your major muscle groups (legs, hips, abdomen, back, arms, chest, shoulders) and to increase your flexibility and balance—all while keeping your heart rate up.

The home circuit has 12 exercises, plus warmup and cooldown: The warmup is performed at an easy pace and prepares your body for low-level aerobic and strength activity. Each exercise, or group of exercises, will require you to move to a different location in your house and keep moving! The cooldown prepares the body for the flexibility exercises and promotes a more relaxed state.

So turn off the TV and crank up some tunes. You'll probably need about six songs (and make your last song a slower tempo).

Do this home circuit consistently three times a week. In a couple of weeks, you should feel your confidence and coordination start to pick up.

Room Setup
Setting up the room beforehand minimizes the chances of accidents and injuries.

- Floors should be nonslip and free of obstructions.
- Weights, water bottles, canned foods, or any other equipment should be placed on a counter.
- Use a straight-back chair without arms. The chair should be high enough to grab the back of.
- Have a kitchen timer or stopwatch at the ready.

Warmup Mountain Pose— Marching

Many physical problems begin with poor posture. You know what it looks like—think of sitting or standing slumped with your head forward and your shoulders rounded. Good posture can strengthen your everyday movements and even make you look taller! Are you aware of your posture? Let's perform an easy Mountain Pose—an ideal postural alignment.

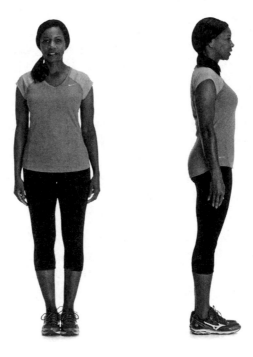

1. Stand with your big toes and ankles together.

2. Drop your tailbone, pulling your belly button inward and upward.

3. With your arms by your sides, relax your shoulders and stand with ears over your shoulders. Drop your chin slightly and gaze ahead.

4. Grow taller by rooting yourself into the ground (nothing lasting can be built on a shaky foundation). Imagine a string pulling you upward, from the top of your head. Good posture is hard work!

5. Now say out loud (or just think it), "I am a strong and resilient woman."

Start marching.

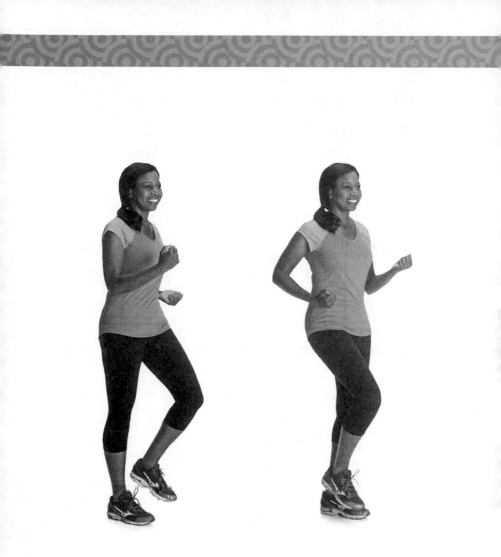

6. Bend your elbows and lightly curl your hands. Swing your arms from your hips to your shoulders as you march. Make sure to keep your elbows close to your body. No chicken wings!

7. Start marching to your favorite upbeat tune. Make sure it's a pace that is slightly challenging and will get your heart rate up after a minute.

8. Do the warmup march for 3 minutes. Feel free to move around the room. March from corner to corner or move forward and backward. Feel gratitude as you catch a glimpse of family photos, or feel inspired as you gather decorating ideas for your family space.

March to the kitchen.

Exercise #1—
Still Arm Hold

(targets shoulders, upper back, and triceps)

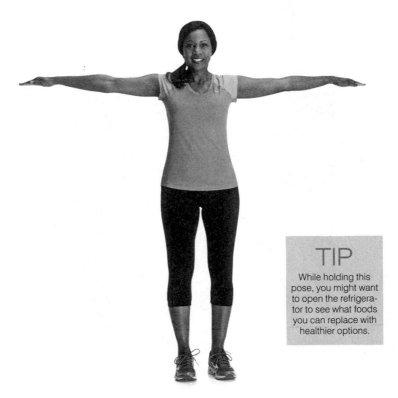

TIP

While holding this pose, you might want to open the refrigerator to see what foods you can replace with healthier options.

1. Stop marching. Stand in Mountain Pose with feet separated hip-width apart—shoulders relaxed, tummy tucked, and eyes straight ahead.

2. Keep your hands at your sides, facing your body.

3. Raise both arms away from your sides like a bird in flight, keeping a slight bend in the elbows and arms no higher than your shoulders. Hold your arms strong (no sagging shoulders!). You should be able to draw a straight line from fingertip to fingertip.

4. Hold this position for 60 seconds. Maintain posture throughout.

March to the bedroom.

Exercise #2—Alternating Kicks
(targets heart, legs, hips, arms, balance, and coordination)

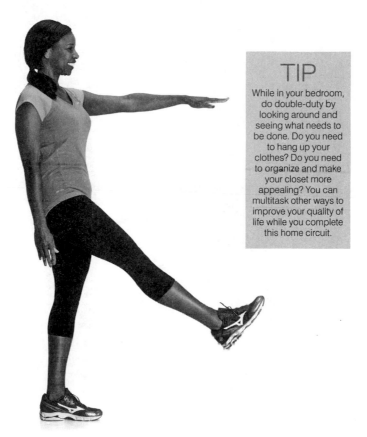

TIP

While in your bedroom, do double-duty by looking around and seeing what needs to be done. Do you need to hang up your clothes? Do you need to organize and make your closet more appealing? You can multitask other ways to improve your quality of life while you complete this home circuit.

1. Stand in mountain pose with your feet hip-width apart, abs tight.

2. Kick your right leg out in front of your body and at the same time raise your left arm.

3. Alternate right leg, left arm–left leg, right arm, keeping legs below the hips as you kick and arms below shoulder height as you reach.

4. Perform for 60 seconds.

March to the living room.

Exercise #3—Butterfly
(targets chest, shoulders, and upper back)

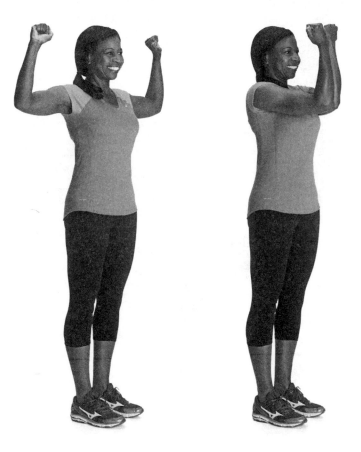

1. Stand in Mountain Pose with feet hip-width apart.

2. Raise arms with your elbows out to the side and palms facing forward. This should look like a goal post.

3. Make a fist and slowly bring your elbows in to touch with knuckles facing away from your face. You should be able to see your manicure.

4. Pause. Then, slowly return to the open goal post position.

5. Perform for 60 seconds, opening and closing.

March to the kitchen.

Exercise #4—Knee Lifts

(targets lower abs and thighs
and challenges balance)

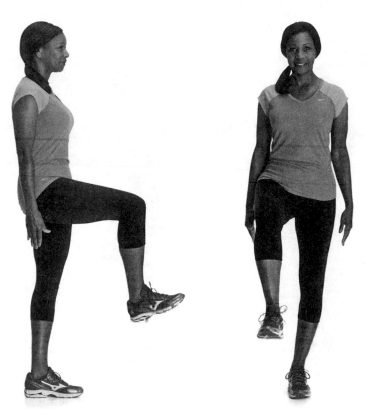

1. Stand at the kitchen counter in Mountain Pose, touching the counter only if you need to balance.

2. Lift your right knee as high as you can, but don't go past your waist. Hold for 5 seconds, then lower it. Alternate knees. Stay tall and keep your abs engaged and hips squared.

3. Perform for 60 seconds.

March back to the living room.

Exercise #5— Arm Reach March
(targets heart, shoulders, arms, and legs)

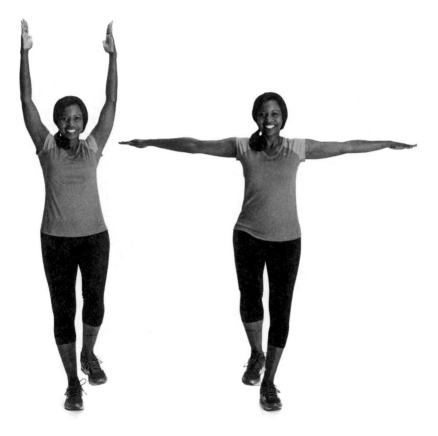

1. March in place.

2. While marching in place reach both arms up toward the ceiling as you draw in your abs.

3. Lower arms to shoulder height and reach out to the sides.

4. Alternate reaching both arms up and out while marching.

5. Perform for 60 seconds.

March to the bedroom.

Exercise #6—Biceps Curl

(targets upper arms)

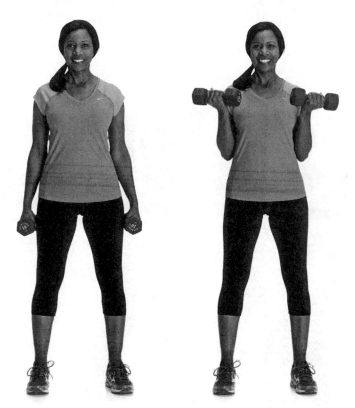

1. Stop marching. Grab light weights, soup cans, or water bottles. (Your weights should be heavy enough so the last few counts make you feel fatigued.)

2. Stand in Mountain Pose with your feet shoulder-width apart and your knees slightly bent and weights in each hand. Hold your arms against your sides with your palms facing inward.

3. Hold your tummy in, and keeping your elbows close to your sides, curl your forearms toward your shoulders so that you can see your manicure. Pause for a second, and then gradually lower your weights back to their starting position.

4. Perform for 60 seconds.

March to the living room.

Exercise #7—
Modified Jumping Jacks
(targets heart, legs, shoulders, abs, and arms)

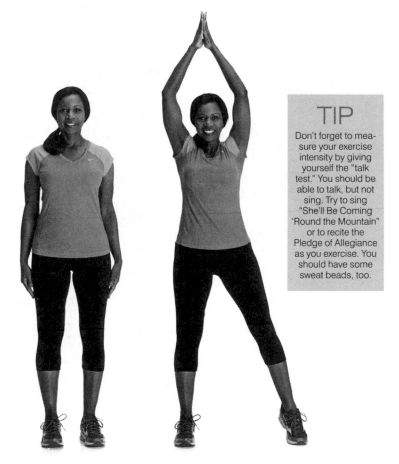

> ### TIP
>
> Don't forget to measure your exercise intensity by giving yourself the "talk test." You should be able to talk, but not sing. Try to sing "She'll Be Coming 'Round the Mountain" or to recite the Pledge of Allegiance as you exercise. You should have some sweat beads, too.

1. Stand in Mountain Pose with feet hip-width apart.

2. Step one foot out to the side and tap. At the same time, raise your arms above your head and clap. Return to the starting position and alternate side to side at a steady pace.

3. Perform for 60 seconds.

March to the dining room.

Exercise #8—Sit and Lean
(targets abs and obliques)

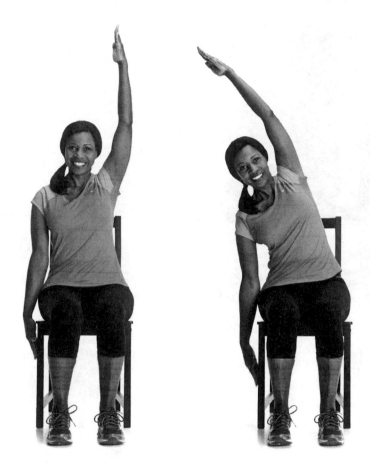

1. Sit on the edge of a chair, feet hip-width apart, with your abs engaged and your shoulders relaxed.

2. Raise your left arm above your head and slowly lean to the right until you feel mild tension on your side. Don't lift your butt from the chair or lean forward or backward. Hold for 30 seconds. Return to the upright position.

3. Switch to the other side. Hold for 30 seconds.

Stay where you are.

Exercise #9—Sit and Stand
(targets legs, abs, and buttocks)

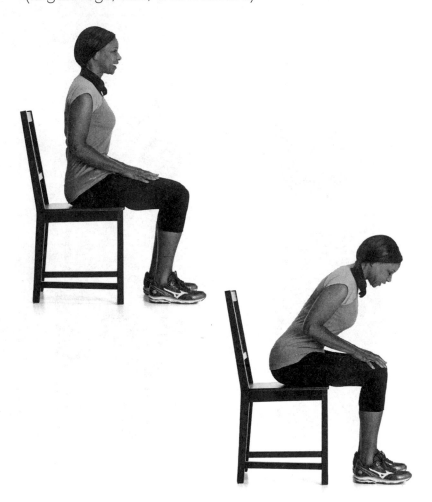

1. Sit in the middle of a sturdy chair without arms.

2. Keep your feet flat on the floor with hands on your thighs closer to your knees.

3. Lean forward, so that your nose is over your toes, then stand up.

4. Bend at your hips and slowly lower your weight down while reaching back with your butt and sit back down.

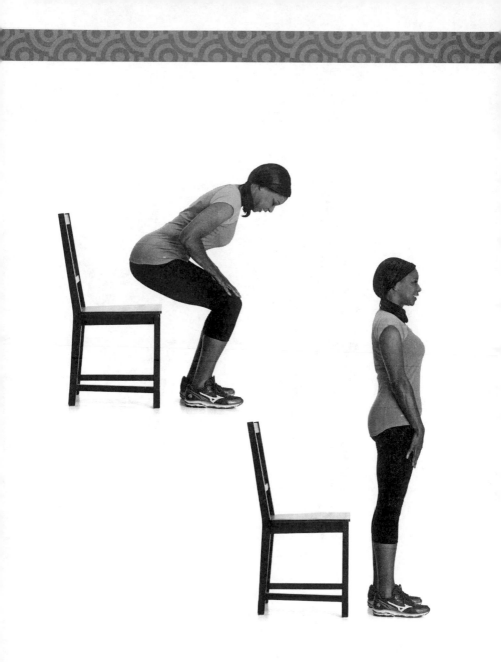

5. Perform for 60 seconds (sit a couple out if needed).

6. Breathe in when standing and breathe out when sitting. Try not to use your hands to assist you.

March to the living room.

Exercise #10—
Jog Easy in Place
(targets heart, legs, and arms)

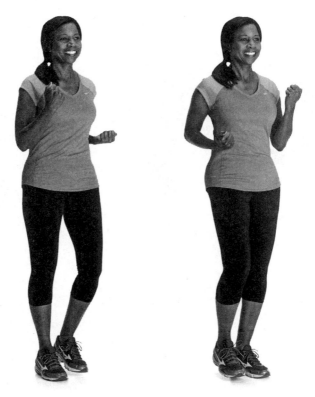

1. Stand tall and walk moderately in place.

2. Move to a quicker speed by lifting your feet only an inch or two off the floor for 20 seconds.

3. Swing your arms from your hips to your shoulders as you jog easy.

4. Alternate 10 seconds of brisk walking and 20 seconds of easy jogging for a total of 60 seconds.

Feel free to walk forward and back or around the couch or wherever your walk takes you. Then walk to the hall.

Exercise #11—Wall Pushups
(targets chest, arms, and shoulders)

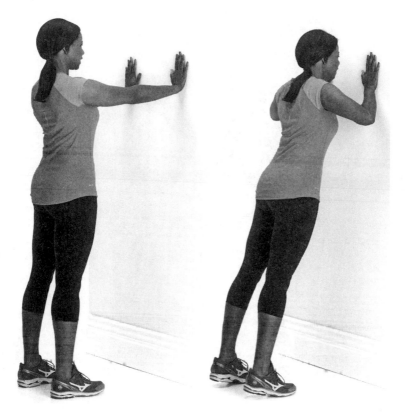

1. Stand facing a wall with your feet slightly apart and your knees slightly bent. Extend your arms in front of you to the wall with your elbows slightly bent. Keep your abs tight.

2. Lean forward slightly and place your palms against the wall. Bend your elbows until your nose nearly touches the wall. Push back out to the starting position. (If it is too hard to get your nose to the wall, go a quarter of the way.)

3. Perform for 60 seconds.

March back to the kitchen.

Exercise #12—
Leg Lifts Abduction
(targets legs, hips, and balance)

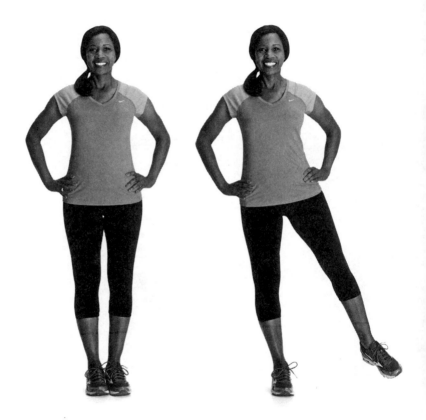

1. Stand in Mountain Pose in front of your kitchen counter with your hands on your hips. Touch only if you need to balance.

2. Raise your left leg out to the side in a smooth movement while balancing on your standing leg, and return. (No leaning to the side; keep abs tight.) Do 10 times on the same leg.

3. Switch legs and continue on the other side.

4. Perform for 60 seconds, switching legs.

For 3 minutes, march slowly to lower your heart rate. (Change your tunes to a slower tempo.)

Quadriceps Stretch

Quad stretches target muscles in the fronts of your thighs. This stretch improves flexibility in your hips, knees, and thigh muscles and helps you run, jump, pedal a bike, or kick a ball.

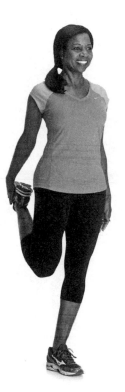

MODIFICATION

Make the stretch easier by placing a chair behind you. Instead of reaching for your ankle with your right hand, bend your right leg until the shin rests on the seat of the chair.

1. Stand up straight behind a chair for balance, with your feet about shoulder-width apart and your knees straight but not locked.

2. Bend your right leg back and grasp your ankle in your right hand. Gently pull your heel up and back toward your butt until you feel light tension in the front of your thigh.

3. Keep the standing leg slightly bent and your hips squared.

4. Tighten your stomach muscles and keep your knees as close together as possible. Breathe throughout the stretch, concentrating on relaxing.

5. Hold for 20 seconds.

6. Repeat the stretch twice on each side, holding for 20 seconds each time.

Hamstring/Calf Stretch

Your hamstring muscle runs along the back of your upper leg and is commonly a tight area, especially for runners and walkers. Stretching your hamstring is important for the health of your back, hips, and knees. Your calf muscle runs along the back of your lower leg. If you wear high heels, calf stretches will keep you in stride.

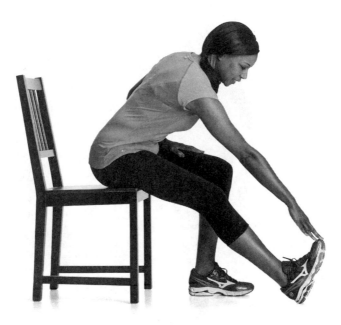

1. Sit on the edge of a chair with your knees bent and feet flat on the floor.

2. Extend your right leg in front of you, placing your right heel on the floor and keeping your ankle relaxed. Don't lock your knee.

3. Slowly lean forward at the hips, reaching for your right toes, trying to keep your back straight and your head lifted.

4. Hold the stretch for a slow count of 20, breathing throughout. Don't push the stretch too far; you should feel the first part of this stretch in the back of the upper leg and the second part in the calf.

5. Switch legs and repeat.

Chest and Arm Stretch

This stretch will improve the flexibility in your arms and chest and in the fronts of your shoulders. It targets a group of muscles particularly vulnerable to tension and stress—the neck, back, and shoulders. You can also do it during any activity that makes you feel stiff, such as sitting at a desk. You'll find it makes you feel young again!

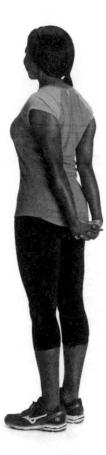

1. Stand with your arms at your sides and your feet slighly apart.

2. Extend both arms behind your back and clasp your hands together, if possible, pulling your shoulders back and extending your arms downward.

3. Hold the stretch for a slow count of 20, breathing throughout.

4. Release the stretch and repeat.

Build Your Own Circuit

Familiarize yourself with the exercises in the circuit and do them for the next 21 days. You can always take your circuit workout outside for new scenery and props. Begin with a walk, jog, or bike ride. For the chairs in Exercise #8 and #9, substitute a series of park benches. Find a wall or a sturdy tree for exercise #11.

You could even add on a few extra variations to your circuit to have fun outside and take things up a notch: Walk up and down steps or a hill, jog backward, or do a side shuffle. Add situps, squats, and walking lunges on the grass, or do pushups and triceps dips on a bench or picnic table. Don't forget to warm up, cool down, and end with flexibility and stretching.

Tracking Your Progress

To help you keep track of your gains, you need to get into the practice of monitoring your work and your progress. A plain old calendar—on your wall or on your computer—is a simple way to log how often you exercise and what type of exercise you do, and will keep you motivated and on track. Use your bathroom scale as a loose gauge to see how well you are keeping on track—just don't get hung up on the numbers! Also, break out the tape measure to see how much your waist circumference is going down. Every little helps a little!

Each day you exercise, reward yourself with a star or smiley face on the calendar. The calendar is a visual reminder of how well you are doing. Another way to keep you motivated and help you reach your goals is a tip jar. If you tip yourself a dollar after each workout, your progress really starts to pay off!

Incorporate more spontaneous physical activity like standing, walking, fidgeting, and shifting while sitting. These movements count, as well.

Eventually, your body will adapt to your exercises and will require new types of exercise to stay challenged. You can modify the intensity of the circuit by jogging instead of marching or by increasing the amount of weight you are using. I see women spending time in my gym working out 3 to 5 days a week without experiencing any change to their physique or measuring their performance. Don't waste your time or effort—you *will* need to kick up your intensity.

Because you have read this far, I believe you have made a commitment to change. To get even more improvements, continue to practice your affirmations and meditations so you can be your own inspiration.

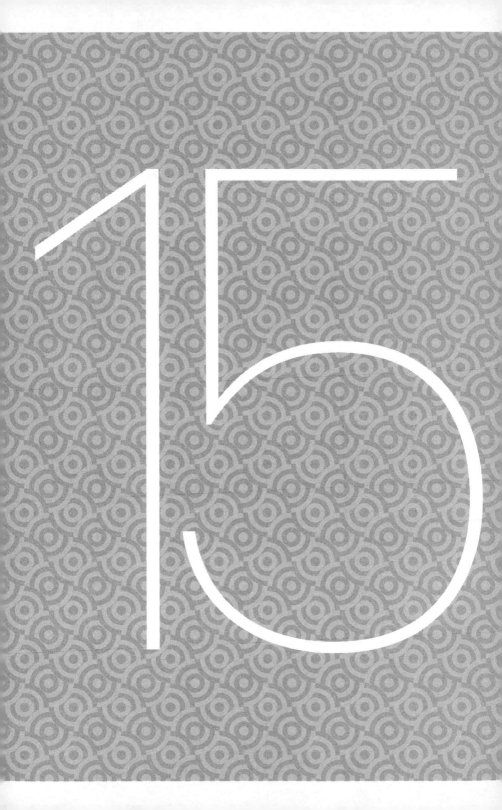

Shaping Up America

Join the Movement

MY TOWN OF VICKSBURG HAPPENS TO BE located in what was for years America's fattest and poorest state, but each community has its own health issues. Maybe you live in a suburban area where everyone drives and there are no sidewalks. Or maybe you live in an urban neighborhood with limited access to fresh food. Regardless, what every community can take away from the Vicksburg experience is the idea that we're all in it together, and this is the key to real change. Everyone needs to take care of his or her own body, but we can help each other achieve our goals.

Lately, the public health focus in this country has centered on how we are going to finance our exploding health-care costs, but far too little attention has been paid to stopping the causes of poor health. Communities, by definition, concern themselves with people. We should share the responsibility with our towns, our states, and the nation for developing ideas for joining together to promote good health.

Obesity has many faces: rich, poor, elderly, young, families, individuals, men, women, those with disabilities, and those without them. We work together, commute together, pray together, celebrate together, and live together. Still, individual circumstances keep us locked in unhealthy lifestyles—overwork, new parenthood, joblessness, caretaking, abusive relationships. I have said over and over again that if we are to turn this obesity epidemic around, we must use the greatest weapon we have: the ability to help each other.

As members of Shape Up Vicksburg's walking club discovered, getting up at dawn for a power walk alone is lonely. But meeting a friend or a group is a celebration. Soon the number of walkers grew and so did the commitment of each member. With friends and neighbors sharing victories and defeats, you feel part of something bigger than yourself, and you push yourself to go further than you thought possible. At the Shape Up Sisters gym, members have the support of many other women who do not let their failures define them. They let their failures teach them, and they let others help pick them up to start again.

A Shape Up community can be a movement of hundreds or as small as five people. You can create a lunchtime walking club at work, share low-calorie recipes with fitness-minded coworkers, or start a Sunday support group at your church. No matter where you are, you are always within range of somebody who would like to get in shape, too. Join forces, and suddenly something that seemed like a chore becomes a pleasure. Something that seemed easy to ignore becomes woven into daily life.

On the national level, First Lady Michelle Obama has truly changed the conversation about the connection between exercise and health, and childhood obesity in particular. Her

Let's Move! initiative started in 2009, about the same time as the Shape Up Vicksburg weight-loss challenge. Because Mississippi has seen a 13 percent decline in childhood obesity since Let's Move! began, a couple of years ago Mrs. Obama visited an elementary school in Clinton, located about 20 minutes from Vicksburg, to promote and celebrate the third anniversary of her initiative. I was fortunate enough to be in the school gym with the First Lady, and I spoke with her about the work being done in Vicksburg. She thanked me, we shook hands, and she joined Rachael Ray in the school cafeteria to prepare school lunches for the children.

"We are seeing there is hope, and when a nation comes together and everyone is thinking about this issue and trying to figure out what role they can play, then we can see change," the First Lady said to journalist Robin Roberts, a native of Mississippi. (Roberts remarked that if Mississippians could fry water, we would!)

When everyone finds a role, the result can be electrifying. We were fortunate to have the media pick up on our efforts in Vicksburg, and after a segment depicting our obesity plight aired on *NBC Nightly News with Brian Williams,* I received a call from a Missouri woman named Christiana. Christiana had seen the segment, which featured Kayla, a 14-year-old girl whose battle with diabetes and being overweight landed her in the hospital and then in my gym. The cameraman had shot a close-up of Kayla's shoes as she was walking on the treadmill. That image of her shoes must have melted Christiana's heart because she immediately called me and said she wanted to buy Kayla a brand new pair of tennis shoes to comfortably work out in. From more than 500 miles away, Christiana's kind, nurturing heart touched us here at Shape Up Sisters.

There are so many ways to get engaged and support others. On the following pages, I have outlined the role you can play in helping to set goals and start improving people's lives in your community, your state, and our nation. What I've learned from doing this is that no one ever starts out equipped with all the skills and knowledge we ultimately will need to accomplish a big goal. But if you have a desire to help, that is the crucial first step. You can also find a ton of useful links and tools to start your own Shape Up movement at LindaFondren.com.

Linda's List for Shaping Up America
Ending Obesity One Community at a Time

Define Your Mission. Why do you want to take this journey? You must examine your own life and find your true purpose before challenging an entire community. Again, get the speck out of your own eye, so you can see clearly and help remove it from someone else's. Why are you really doing this? Why take the risk—and the time—to make changes? The most important word here is "Why."

Your mission will guide your actions. My mission took hold after the death of my sister. I developed a strong desire to give obese and overweight women a chance at a better quality of life by helping them become more active and lose weight. I learned by doing, and the desire to help women led to the desire to help a wider population, especially those who lack the resources to achieve a healthy lifestyle. Desire is the starting point that leads to the mission, and for me it was the reason I wrote this book.

Patrick House, a fellow Vicksburg resident, is an inspiring example of someone who defined his mission clearly. Patrick was the first Mississippian to be on the hit NBC series *The Biggest Loser,* and he was the show's winner for Season 10. Patrick says he went on the show so that he could enjoy a better life with his wife and young children. He wanted to be the dad who could chase his son around the yard or ride on roller-coasters, but because he tipped the scales at 400 pounds, that was impossible. "When I look back, especially growing up, life revolved around food and fellowship," Patrick says. "Food is a lot of people's main comfort. They might not have a lot of money for a lot of things, but they can always cook you a great meal. My mom makes a mean green bean casserole!"

After shedding 181 pounds in the weight-loss contest, Patrick has remained fit and set out to become a role model to thousands of Mississippians. He authored a book, *As Big as a House,* and began the Lean on Me program, where he goes to elementary schools throughout the state to educate young children on nutrition, health, and standing up for themselves in the face of bullying.

Patrick and I have often joined forces to promote nutrition and exercise, and I see him as a force for change. "I truly believe Mississippi has turned a corner," Patrick says. With people like him committed to inspiring others, we can't go wrong.

Set a Precise Goal (or Set of Goals). You must transform your mission into a doable goal or goals so you know exactly what you aim to accomplish. The wording of your goal should be clear. Remember the definition of a workable goal I gave you in Chapter 9? A goal should be something that stretches you but that you feel you can attain. My mission was to give obese and overweight Vicksburg residents a new chance at life, and my goal was to have them collectively lose 17,000 pounds in 17 weeks.

Ultimately, as you know, we did not reach that goal. But along the way we met several other short-term goals. Not only did we collectively lose 15,000 pounds, but we realized there was a need to accomplish a separate (but related) goal of helping teens improve their eating habits, for which we would need to take a different approach. Designed by the state Office of Women's Health, Bodyworks became a 4- to 8-week program offering Shape Up Vicksburg parents the tools to help their teens learn to eat better, start to exercise, and maintain a healthy weight. It was a perfect complement to our original goal. At every session, women reported back about a small step they had taken to help change their family's eating and exercise habits.

Your short-term goals will change as you progress and learn more. Stay flexible and open-minded and you will achieve more than you ever dreamed of.

Assess Your Community. The places where we live, work, learn, worship, and play shape and define the choices we make—and, in turn, our health. A healthy community develops when healthy lifestyle choices are incorporated seamlessly into everyday life.

What aspects of your community are in greatest need of improvement to help promote the health of all citizens? What are the obstacles your community faces to more physical activity and healthy eating? What are some of the root causes of these problems—poverty, lack of motivation, poor housing conditions, high unemployment, high crime rates, physical inactivity, or limited access to healthy foods and affordable health care? Poverty can be defined by income level, but it doesn't necessarily define the conditions people really live in. In other words, are the individuals in your neighborhood in a position to improve their lives? The problem may not lie with the whole community, but with certain neighborhoods or populations.

Successful planning requires deep knowledge of your community. Otherwise, you could impose intervention strategies that are ineffective and miss opportunities for attainable goals. For instance, at one point I proposed a goal to our local elected officials to ban smoking on city- and county-owned properties. However, I encountered huge resistance. "That would be an invasion of privacy!" they crowed. "It's people's right to do things to harm their health." And my favorite: "You can't ban smoking on public golf courses!"

The no-smoking ban was the kind of goal that might have been more effective if I'd started by gauging interest from residents and gathering signatures in a petition before bringing the idea to elected officials. My advice: Take time to get to know the population you are trying to help and the decision makers who will be assisting you.

Develop a Strategy. Break down the steps you must take to achieve your goal. Does your goal focus on children, adults, infrastructure, services, or all of the above? Determine what you need, who can help you get what you need, how to ask for what you need, and who—if not you—will do it. To make the most of your time and resources, consider the best place to start. How will you get people to change their behaviors? How will you pay for your program? How will you communicate your efforts? How will you measure the outcome of your actions? The key word here is "How."

Take Action. Once you have defined your mission, set your goals, assessed your community, and developed a strategy, then it's time to take action. You've spent a lot of time and effort figuring out what needs to be done, so now do it. Execute your plan, and even if you have to revise it later, don't get bogged down in analysis that might paralyze you from moving forward.

Come Up with Metrics to Determine Success. There is no real evidence of success without measurements. I'm talking about data. Are you just doing a good deed or helping to shape up your community in concrete ways? For Shape Up Vicksburg, we put a weight loss log on our Web site so participants could create their own accounts and record their weight loss. We installed weigh-in stations at various businesses and scales that measured weight and body composition. We were able to see where we were at every stage of our challenge, which motivated us to try harder.

Other metrics we used to measure success included attendance at walk programs (we always wanted those numbers to increase!), Likes on Facebook, new applications to join the walking club, and attendance in the gym on Saturday, which is when it's open to the public for free.

All of these metrics will come in handy when people

ask—and they will—"Hey, how's it going?" You will be able to point to these different areas of progress. Seeing concrete data on how you're doing with your effort can also help you refine your strategies (if it's not working, try something else!), hone your communication, or rethink your finances so you can meet the goal you've set for yourself.

Develop Strategic Partnerships. Are other groups already doing something like what you want to do or have a way of communicating to the audience you are looking to reach? You may be able to link up with another national, state, or local organization, especially if you have problems (funding or otherwise) getting your mission off the ground. Partnerships are an important option to help your mission.

One of the first places to check if you're trying to start a community fitness program is the Web site for Healthy Parks, Healthy People US (www.nps.gov/public_health/hp/hphp.htm). This initiative reaches residents who traditionally have not participated in park programming and promotes the health benefits of exploring our public parks. It's a fact that people tend to exercise longer when they take it outdoors. One of my favorite places to play when I was a kid was on the monuments of the Vicksburg National Military Park. Growing up in poverty meant lots of opportunities for creative, outdoor physical activity, and I would race up and down the 47 steps of the Illinois monument, one for each day of the siege of Vicksburg during the Civil War, and slide on a piece of cardboard down those big grassy hills lined by cannons.

Our national park has been a huge part of the Shape Up Vicksburg initiative, and the way it came about may be instructive. When we were starting out, I was surprised when the superintendent of the park asked me point blank, "Why do so few African Americans walk in the park?" I knew it was because the black community felt uncomfortable in areas that glorify the history of the Confederacy. I also told him truthfully that exercise is at the bottom of a long list of priorities for many blacks, and that's what I was trying to change.

Since then, First Lady Michelle Obama designated the Vicksburg National Military Park as a "Let's Move Outside" park—a place for families to get healthy and stay fit. The huge, 1,728-acre park has 12.5 miles of walking trails, 16 miles of tour roads, and 1,325 historic monuments, markers, and plaques. A couple of years ago, Shape Up Vicksburg and the park teamed up to hash out ideas about how to change blacks' perceptions of this Civil War park. We wanted to get everyone to view the monuments of the park as art, the scenery as nature, and the history as a narrative of restored self-respect. And we wanted to get people to use the park for physical activity. So the park agreed to waive the entrance fee and promoted use of the area during Black History Month under the theme Our Shared History, Our Shared Community, Our Shared Health.

Since Black History Month falls in February, we thought the weather might keep people away. But hundreds of first timers came, and people continue to come for the walks each year. Blacks and whites walk together for up to 3 miles on a path that takes them by the park's greatest historical spots: the United States Colored Troop Monument, representing African American men who served in armies of both the Union and Confederacy; the USS *Cairo*, on which African American sailors served with whites to take on the Confederates (the ship was sunk in 1862 with no casualties); the place where activist Medgar Evers gave his civil rights speech and courted his wife, Myrlie; and Beulah Cemetery, which dates to 1884 and is the oldest resting place of many former leaders of Vicksburg's African American community. At each spot, the National Park Service staff is present to welcome walkers and interpret the history of the park.

Shape Up Vicksburg also joined with city agencies to create a walking trail for mothers to use while their children take swimming lessons and play in the skate park. We partnered with the Vicksburg Rotary Club for a bike safety seminar and an educational bike tour in parts of the Vicksburg National Military Park. And we became a sponsor of major walking and running events, like Over the River Run and Chill in the Hills, to give residents a chance to participate in a major race at no cost. We joined forces with Let's Go Walkin' Mississippi—a statewide walking program—as well as Alcorn State University, AmeriCorps, and several local schools and public health organizations. Community partners can also be an important resource for grant funding.

Plan Your Finances. Know what your resources are, come up with a budget, keep good records, don't overextend yourself, and look around for grants. Applying for nonprofit status can make you eligible for all sorts of grants from private corporations and foundations looking to underwrite health and educational initiatives. Partnerships can come in handy here—sometimes it's easier to win a grant when you team up with another group. For instance, the Vicksburg National Military Park and Shape Up Vicksburg applied for and received a grant to create the Shape Up Junior Ranger program for 6- to 12-year-olds. Each recruit received a Shape Up Junior Ranger logbook, a "fit kit" with a pedometer, and a water bottle and backpack donated by Walgreens.

Finally, I strongly recommend the book *The Art of Doing Good: Where Passion Meets Action,* by Charles Bronfman and Jeffrey Solomon. It tackles how you grow from an idea to a program or movement, with advice for launching a nonprofit. Reading about how others have succeeded can help you be more effective.

Become Involved in Community Development. Playing an active role in community development in your city and state can promote healthy lifestyles by directing attention and resources toward planning sidewalks, farmers' markets, and playgrounds. A community assessment enables you to become familiar with your area's history, geography, and political leadership. This knowledge allows you to develop personal relationships and build trust. Reaching out lets you get involved in the community activities of schools, churches, civic clubs, chambers of commerce, and cultural and art organizations. Keep in mind that some of the most important information about your community may be hidden in the underserved community.

Again, you may find that good social programs already exist in your town or city. Instead of duplicating what is already being done, see how you can leverage these efforts and then extend beyond them.

Use the Media as a Resource and a Bullhorn. The media influences what issues we think about and how we think about them, particularly decisions pertaining to our personal health and health policy. You can turn to traditional local media—like print, television, or radio—and new social media— like Twitter and Facebook—to amplify your voice. The media has an enormous capacity to reach and educate people, and educated people are less likely to be obese, smoke, or engage in other unhealthy habits.

Before you try to communicate anything, be very clear about your message. You typically have one chance to pitch your idea, so make sure you can sum it up in a few words and are clear about its benefit to the public. Take the time to develop a positive relationship with your local media outlets, like the local newspaper or radio station. It doesn't have to be complicated—just go into their offices and introduce yourself. Shake hands. It will be worth it in the long run.

Empower the People You're Trying to Help. One of the biggest obstacles to success will be the motivation and commitment of the very public you are aiming to reach. Even with benefits like free access to gyms or nutritional education, making sustainable lifestyle changes is very difficult.

Involve your community in the action by giving individuals or groups a stake in spreading the message. For instance, in our 4-week Bodyworks program for teens, we empowered teachers to become Role Models for Students. On Workout Wednesdays, teachers wore their workout clothes to school and set an example by eating healthy lunches and attending workout classes with the kids. For another program, called Operation

Empowerment, we reached out to female heads of households in the underserved community who could role-model our program, in which we took them to doctors for checkups, supported them while getting their GED, and provided them with toolkits for changing habits such as cookbooks, pedometers, and fitness journals. These women were able to lead by example with the tools we gave them, and they spread the example of healthy living across their circles. They could share knowledge on nutrition, exercise, and lifestyle with others to help break the cycle of obesity that is killing our community.

Trust and Be Trusted. Communities face so many hardships. Your mission to help people in the community adopt healthier behaviors is noble, but no program will suddenly erase discrimination or eliminate distrust carried over from bad experiences. Your program will have to work to instill the belief that not only do individuals have the ability to change their own lives, but they can also influence their community at large.

Building trust was crucial in the early days of our challenge. To boost enrollment in Shape Up Vicksburg, I visited neighborhoods where people sat on their porches while kids played outside. I approached one woman who sat by her door in a sagging lawn chair that was threatening to collapse as her 2-year-old son roamed around the yard. She was clearly apprehensive about two strangers approaching her property.

"What you want?!" she yelled at us.

My volunteer handed the woman a flier and went into the pitch about our 6-week nutrition and exercise program. To this woman, however, talk was cheap. The woman read through the flier and hammered us with questions, "Who is this for?" "How much it cost?" "Why are you doing this?" "Do I need it?" All were good questions. As we answered each question, I could see her wrestling with the idea that there was something specifically designed for her. She could not believe anyone would see value in *her*.

I knew for a fact that she could change, and I wanted to

give her a way to change. When we left, I wasn't sure I would see her again, but I was sure that we would keep being persistent. I thought, she'll hear our message if we keep on saying it.

Well, guess who showed up on day one with her baby in tow? That's right. She was still apprehensive, still doubtful, but she was there. She took the first step because we did not give up on her. I knew one of the most important things we could do for this woman's son was to provide her with an opportunity to get healthy.

Leverage the Skills of Others. To maximize your effectiveness and broaden your knowledge base, you need to work with elected officials, doctors, health educators, nurses, clinical psychologists, social workers, dietitians, hospitals, colleges, schools, churches, farmers' markets, policemen, firemen, civic clubs, childcare centers, walking clubs, and others to supplement the skills you don't have.

Be Patient and Be Tireless. Success rarely happens right away. It will take many face-to-face meetings with community members and officials, skilled use of social media, and group committee meetings. Effective connections with partners and elected officials will help you convince others of the value and importance of your idea. And even once you have all of that in place, mobilizing a large population and seeing measurable results all take time.

This is something everyone can do. Around the country, we are just beginning to focus on the fact that the health of our communities and our personal health are deeply connected. To thrive, we need an inclusive economic vision that helps people to help themselves—and others.

I hope that the journey I've taken you on through this book, from my own beginnings to what we have created in Vicksburg, gives you a picture of what is possible. With highly motivated individuals like you shaping up healthy communities across America, the future looks extremely bright.

Epilogue

Something I Have to Do

HAVE YOU WONDERED IF SOMEONE YOU love was looking down on you from above, smiling? When my sister Mary passed on to heaven in 2006, she had no idea that the comments she made to me on her deathbed—wishing she had lived her life more for herself—would become my motivating purpose, one that would ultimately lead me to write this book. She had no idea I would open a gym called Shape Up Sisters to help women like her who wanted to change but lacked the confidence and know-how to do so. She had no idea her true confession would spur a movement called Shape Up Vicksburg and help a community lose 15,000 pounds. She only knew she needed to get something off her chest before she passed.

I, too, must confess something. Some years before I began writing *Shape Up Sisters,* I had started writing another book, a memoir about my rags-to-riches life experience. But that book got sidelined when I returned to Mississippi. My homecoming brought confusion to my heart and my brain. I saw that not much had changed for women. Households led by single mothers, poverty, obesity, teenage pregnancy, ignorance, racism, lack of good role models, lack of self-esteem, and a host of others factors still kept so many locked in unhealthy lifestyles.

I made it out of that life, but I thought that how I did that was not the story I should try to tell. My desire was to help the community and not embarrass my family and friends with my connection to prostitution. Even though what I did was perfectly legal, I knew the stigma still remained. I didn't want to shatter the trust of the people who now saw me and my success as a bright light of hope. So, that memoir sat in a drawer.

But I burned with the need to say something to help people, especially women. This burning need to do *something* guided me on a mission to write a book focused on obesity prevention, to help women with struggles more similar to my sister's than to my own.

But, as they say, if you want to make God laugh, tell him your plans. In the course of working on the book about obesity, I decided to run for mayor of Vicksburg. I had no illusions about the political process, and I realized parts of my past would probably come to light and be distorted to paint me as an undesirable candidate. And I was right. But a funny thing happened: Rather than reject or judge me, the vast majority of folks seemed to embrace my story, and me. People told me that they felt they had more in common with me now that they knew some of the struggles in my life. While I came in second in the race, I felt that I had won something more precious: a deeper connection to the people of my community. I realized that the book I was trying to write about stemming the tide of obesity was not just for people like my sister, it was for me—it was for all of us who need empowerment to create a healthy, vibrant, meaningful life. Although I am not obese, the story of how I created change for myself that eventually led to a happy, healthy life full of purpose was an important part of the message. Fat is a symptom of deeper things that need changing. Not all of the things that need changing are within our individual control, but when we make a commitment to do better for ourselves and then come together to help each other in our commitments, mountains can be moved.

Time has taught me a powerful lesson: I have no control over the past or the future, but I can make choices in the present. Some of the best advice I've learned along the way is to say "thank you" rather than get defensive when someone tells me bad news about myself. They have just given me valuable information—either it is information I need to make myself better or it is information about them and how they judge people. Either way, it's useful to know. I have learned to promise nothing, but simply to roll up my sleeves and do what needs to be done. I learned to answer the question, "Why are you doing that?" by simply saying, "It is something I have to do." Don't bother trying to explain your reasons—in fact, as you go toward a goal, your reasons for doing it might change. What remains is the *choice* to do it—that is the one thing that is always consistent. *It is something I have to do.*

Please believe this: The most powerful way to create the life you want is to tell yourself, and to tell others, that you are blessed beyond your imagination. Your body will become an expression of that radiance. Let your first thought when you wake be about *good health.* Good health is something you have to strive for.

This is not the book I thought I would write. It is the book I had to write. I think Mary is smiling right now. Every day of your life is a chapter in *your* book.

Acknowledgments

This book would not be possible without the many strong and resilient women I met in my community, both throughout the citywide Shape Up Vicksburg Weight Loss Challenge and my loyal Shape Up Sisters members. They offered their stories of victories and hardships and inspired me every day. Women I met all over the country have generously and humbly shared themselves and their experiences, and I learned and grew through our interactions.

Much gratitude goes to my publisher, Rodale Books, whose staff has patiently and diligently helped me with the process of production, promotion, and perfection. I am particularly grateful to Alex Postman for her editing wisdom, making sure we got it right and helping this book sing to its audience.

I cannot say enough thank-yous to my friend, teacher, and editor Samantha Dunn, who is a master at helping to organize and shape my words to give them more power and clarity. We spent many a late night and early morning gearing up for and finalizing each chapter, line by line. Sam, you are amazing. Thank you for your belief and commitment to the message. You are the kind of girl who climbs the ladder and is not afraid of heights.

Thank you to my agent, Lynn Johnston, for your

razor-sharp mind. You paved the path, helping prepare me for the journey of this book.

I cannot say enough adoring words about Linnie Wheeless, my amazing, analytical friend and assistant. You have contributed to my mission on all levels, and I don't know what I would have done without you. You have embraced impossible missions, opened my mind, and won my heart. I am indebted.

I have been blessed with Rebecca Turner, a busy mom, nutrition expert, and passionate runner. Your deep knowledge was key in helping us to offer more authoritative advice for a healthy, balanced diet.

A heartfelt thanks to my BFF Cindy Gittleman for her continuous support, critiques, and encouragement. I am incredibly grateful for our friendship.

Thank you Values.com, "The Foundation for a Better Life," who shaped my story to help inspire the world! No matter where we live, we live by values. And values are worth more when we pass them on!

I have been fortunate to have an international network like CNN recognize me as a Top 10 CNN Hero. They have contributed greatly in helping the organization grow and sustain our important work. Thank you, CNN and Anderson Cooper.

To my daughter, Chris, and my granddaughter, Kyla: Thanks for keeping me humble and reminding me of the blessings of being a mother and grandmother. To my wonderful and colorful family, thank you for loving me and for supporting me in every endeavor and project I have attempted. Your enthusiastic support and love have been present at all times. Especially thanks to Pat, who always had my back.

And to my dear husband Jim, who believed in me before I believed in myself. No words can convey how much I love and appreciate you, but hopefully, our 29 years of marriage is a start. I am everything I am because you loved me.

Recipes

For Southerners, food is a way of life. It affords us a sense of pride, community, and heritage. Family recipes are time-honored traditions that become ingrained in our memories. Hours are spent at social events and around the kitchen table, and when we're far from home, most of us dream about our favorite dishes.

Most believe that eating traditional Southern cuisine makes you fat, but it doesn't have to be that way. We've already reviewed a number of tricks to make over most any recipe with healthier ingredients (see Chapter 13). In the following pages, you'll find 21 recipes that represent good-for-you versions of many Southern favorites, from Crispy Oven-Fried Chicken to Smothered Greens and Candied Yams. While these are all lower in fat than the originals and are more nutrient-dense, don't forget you still need to be mindful of portion control to keep calories in check.

Now let's get cooking!

Recipe Sources: National Heart, Lung, and Blood Institute; National Institutes of Health; and U.S. Department of Health and Human Services.

Breakfast

Oatmeal Pecan Waffles (or Pancakes)

Cook time: 30 minutes   **Yield:** 4 servings

- 1 cup whole-wheat flour
- ½ cup quick-cooking oats
- 2 teaspoons baking powder
- 1 teaspoon sugar
- ¼ cup unsalted pecans, chopped
- 2 large eggs, separated (for pancakes, see tip)
- 1½ cups fat-free milk
- 1 tablespoon vegetable oil

Fruit Topping

- 2 cups fresh strawberries, rinsed, stems removed, and cut in half (or substitute frozen strawberries, thawed)
- 1 cup fresh blackberries, rinsed (or substitute frozen blackberries, thawed)
- 1 cup fresh blueberries, rinsed (or substitute frozen blueberries, thawed)
- 1 teaspoon powdered sugar

Preheat a waffle iron.

In a big bowl combine the flour, oats, baking powder, sugar, and pecans.

In a separate medium bowl combine the egg yolks, milk, and vegetable oil. Mix well.

Add the liquid mixture to the dry ingredients and stir together. Do not overmix; the mixture should be a bit lumpy.

Whip the egg whites to medium peaks. Gently fold the egg whites into the batter (for pancakes, see the note below).

Pour the batter into the preheated waffle iron and cook until the waffle iron light signals it's done or steam stops coming out of the iron. (A waffle is perfect when it is crisp and well-browned on the outside with a moist, light, airy, and fluffy inside). Or make pancakes.

Add fresh fruit and a light dusting of powdered sugar to each waffle, and serve.

TIP. For pancakes, do not separate the eggs. Mix the whole eggs with the milk and oil, and skip whipping the egg whites.

Summer Breeze Smoothie

Cook time: 0 minutes   **Yield:** 3 servings

1	cup plain nonfat yogurt
6	medium strawberries
1	cup canned crushed pineapple
1	medium banana
1	teaspoon vanilla extract
4	ice cubes

Place all ingredients in a blender and puree until smooth. Serve in a frosted glass.

Main Dishes

Spicy Southern Barbecued Chicken

Cook time: 2 hours   **Yield:** 6 servings

5	tablespoons tomato paste
1	teaspoon ketchup
2	teaspoons honey
1	teaspoon molasses
1	teaspoon Worcestershire sauce
4	teaspoons white vinegar
¾	teaspoon cayenne pepper
⅙	teaspoon black pepper
¼	teaspoon onion powder
2	cloves garlic
⅙	teaspoon grated ginger
1½	pounds skinless chicken (breasts, drumsticks)

Combine all ingredients except the chicken in a saucepan. Simmer for 15 minutes. Wash the chicken and pat dry. Place it on large platter and brush with half the sauce mixture. Cover with plastic wrap and marinate in the refrigerator for 1 hour.

Place the chicken on a baking sheet lined with aluminum foil and broil for 10 minutes on each side to seal in the juices. Remove from the broiler and add the remaining sauce to the chicken. Cover with aluminum foil and bake at 350°F for 30 minutes.

Crispy Oven-Fried Chicken

Cook time: 60–80 minutes   **Yield:** 6 servings

- ½ cup fat-free milk or buttermilk
- 1 teaspoon poultry seasoning
- 1 cup cornflakes, crumbled
- 1½ tablespoons onion powder
- 1½ tablespoons garlic powder
- 2 teaspoons black pepper
- 2 teaspoons dried hot pepper, crushed
- 1 teaspoon ground ginger
- 8 pieces skinless chicken (4 breasts, 4 drumsticks)
- 1 teaspoon vegetable oil
-   A few shakes paprika

Preheat the oven to 350°F. In a small bowl, combine the milk and ½ teaspoon of poultry seasoning.

Combine the cornflake crumbs with all other spices and place in a plastic bag.

Wash the chicken and pat dry. Dip the chicken into the milk and shake to remove excess liquid. Quickly shake it in the bag with the seasonings and crumbs, and remove the chicken from the bag. Refrigerate the chicken for 1 hour. Remove the chicken from the refrigerator and sprinkle it lightly with paprika for color. Space chicken evenly on a baking pan greased with the vegetable oil. Cover with aluminum foil and bake, unturned, for 40 minutes. Remove the foil and continue baking, unturned, for another 30 to 40 minutes or until the meat can easily be pulled away from the bone with a fork. Drumsticks may require less baking time than breasts. Crumbs will form a crispy "skin."

20-Minute Chicken Creole

Cook time: 15 minutes   **Yield:** 4 servings

- 12 ounces boneless, skinless chicken breast, cut into thin strips
- 1 cup canned whole peeled tomatoes, chopped
- 1 cup chili sauce (look for lowest-sodium version)
- 1½ cups chopped green bell pepper
- 1½ cups chopped celery
- ¼ cup chopped onion
- 1 tablespoon minced garlic
- 1 tablespoon fresh basil, rinsed, dried, and chopped (or 1 teaspoon dried)
- 1 tablespoon fresh parsley, rinsed, dried, and chopped (or 1 teaspoon dried)
- ¼ teaspoon crushed red pepper
- ¼ teaspoon salt
  Cooking spray

Spray a sauté pan with cooking spray. Preheat over high heat. Cook the chicken in the hot sauté pan, stirring for 3 to 5 minutes. Reduce the heat. Add the tomatoes with juice, chili sauce, green pepper, celery, onion, garlic, basil, parsley, crushed red pepper, and salt. Bring to a boil over high heat, and then reduce to simmer. Simmer, covered, for 10 minutes.

TIP. Delicious served over rice.

Cornbread-Crusted Turkey

Cook time: 20 minutes   **Yield:** 4 servings

- 1 cup low-fat buttermilk
- 1 tablespoon Dijon mustard
- 4 skinless turkey fillets (3 ounces each)
- 4 -by-4" square prepared cornbread (about 1 cup crumbs) (See Good-for-You Cornbread, page 216)
- 1 egg white (or substitute liquid egg white)
- 1 cup low-sodium chicken broth
- 1 tablespoon cornstarch
- 1 pound frozen baby carrots
- 1 tablespoon fresh sage, rinsed, dried, and chopped (or 1 teaspoon dried)
- 1 tablespoon butter

Preheat the oven to 350°F.

In a small bowl, combine the buttermilk and Dijon mustard. Mix well. Add the turkey fillets to the buttermilk mixture to marinate for 5 to 10 minutes while preparing the cornbread.

Grind the cornbread in a food processor, or use your fingers to make coarse crumbs. Place the bread crumbs on a baking sheet, and dry in a 300°F oven or toaster oven for 4 to 5 minutes. Do not brown. Pour the bread crumbs into a dry, shallow dish. Put the egg white in a separate bowl.

Remove the turkey from the buttermilk and dip each fillet first in the egg white and then in the cornbread crumbs to coat. Be sure to discard the leftover buttermilk mixture and cornbread crumbs.

Place the breaded turkey fillets on a baking sheet, and bake for 10 to 15 minutes (to a minimum internal temperature of 165°F). While the turkey is cooking, combine the chicken broth, cornstarch, carrots, sage, and butter in a medium saucepan. Bring to a boil over high heat, stirring occasionally. Lower the temperature to a simmer. Simmer gently for about 5 minutes, or until the butter is melted, the sauce is thick, and the carrots are warm.

Serve each 3-ounce turkey fillet with 1 cup carrots and sauce mixture.

TIP: Try serving with a baked or roasted sweet potato.

Baked Pork Chops

Cook time: 35 minutes   **Yield:** 6 servings

- 6 lean center-cut pork chops, ½" thick
- 1 egg white
- 1 cup fat-free evaporated milk
- ¾ cup cornflake crumbs
- ¼ cup fine, dry bread crumbs
- 4 teaspoons paprika
- 2 teaspoons oregano
- ¾ teaspoon chili powder
- 2 teaspoons garlic powder
- 2 teaspoons black pepper
- ½ teaspoon cayenne pepper
- ½ teaspoon dry mustard
- 2 teaspoons salt
- Nonstick cooking spray, as needed

Preheat the oven to 375°F.

Trim the fat from the pork chops.

In a small bowl, the beat egg white with the evaporated milk. Place the pork chops in the milk mixture and let stand for 5 minutes, turning once.

Meanwhile, mix the cornflake crumbs, bread crumbs, spices, and salt in a separate small bowl.

Using nonstick cooking spray, coat a 13" x 9" baking pan.

Remove the pork chops from the milk mixture and coat thoroughly with the crumb mixture. Place the pork chops in the coated pan and bake for 20 minutes. Turn the pork chops and bake for an additional 15 minutes or until no pink remains.

NOTE. Try the recipe with skinless, boneless chicken or turkey parts or fish—bake for just 20 minutes.

Mouthwatering Oven-Fried Fish

Cook time: 20 minutes   **Yield:** 6 servings

- 2 pounds fish fillets
- 1 tablespoon fresh lemon juice
- ¼ cup fat-free or 1% buttermilk
- 2 drops hot sauce
- 1 teaspoon minced fresh garlic
- ¼ teaspoon ground white pepper
- ¼ teaspoon salt
- ¼ teaspoon onion powder
- ½ cup crumbled cornflakes or regular bread crumbs
- 1 tablespoon vegetable oil
- 1 fresh lemon, cut in wedges

Preheat the oven to 475°F. Clean and rinse the fish. Wipe the fillets with the lemon juice and pat dry. In a small bowl, combine the milk, hot sauce, and garlic.

In a separate bowl, combine the pepper, salt, and onion powder with the crumbs and spread on a large plate.

Let the fillets sit briefly in the milk. Remove and coat the fillets on both sides with the seasoned crumbs. Let stand briefly until the coating sticks to each side of the fish. Arrange the coated fish on a lightly oiled shallow baking dish. Bake for 20 minutes on the middle rack without turning.

Cut into 6 pieces. Serve with fresh lemon.

Scrumptious Meat Loaf

Cook time: 62 minutes   **Yield:** 6 servings

1	pound extra-lean ground beef
½	cup tomato paste
4	cups chopped onion
4	cups chopped green pepper
1	cup chopped red pepper
1	cup chopped fresh tomatoes, blanched
2	teaspoons low-sodium mustard
4	teaspoons ground black pepper
2	teaspoons chopped hot pepper
2	cloves garlic, chopped
2	scallions, chopped
2	teaspoons ground ginger
8	teaspoons ground nutmeg
1	teaspoon grated orange rind
2	teaspoons crushed thyme
4	cups finely grated bread crumbs

Preheat the oven to 350°F.

Mix all the ingredients together in a large bowl. Place in a 1-pound loaf pan (preferably with a drip rack) and bake, covered, for 50 minutes. Uncover the pan and continue baking for 12 minutes.

Sides

Classic Macaroni and Cheese

Cook time: 35 minutes   **Yield:** 8 servings

2	cups macaroni
2	cups chopped onion
2	cups fat-free evaporated milk
1	medium egg, beaten
¼	teaspoon black pepper
1¼	cups finely shredded low-fat Cheddar cheese
	Nonstick cooking spray, as needed

Cook the macaroni according to directions—but do not add salt to the cooking water. Drain and set aside.

Spray a casserole dish with nonstick cooking spray.

Preheat the oven to 350°F.

Lightly spray a saucepan with nonstick cooking spray. Add the onion and cook for 3 to 4 minutes, or until tender.

In a medium bowl, combine the cooked macaroni, onion, and the rest of the ingredients and mix thoroughly. Transfer the mixture to a casserole dish. Bake for 25 minutes or until bubbly. Let stand for 10 minutes before serving.

Vegetable Stew

Cook time: 35 minutes   **Yield:** 8 servings

- 3 cups water
- 1 cube low-sodium vegetable bouillon
- 2 cups white potatoes, cut into 2" strips
- 2 cups sliced carrots
- 4 cups summer squash, cut into 1" squares
- 1 cup summer squash, cut into 4 chunks
- 1 15-ounce can sweet corn, rinsed and drained (or 2 ears fresh corn, 1½ cups)
- 1 teaspoon thyme
- 2 cloves garlic, minced
- 1 stalk scallion, chopped
- ½ small hot pepper, chopped
- 1 cup coarsely chopped onion
- 1 cup diced tomatoes

Put the water and bouillon in a large pot and bring to a boil. Add the potatoes and carrots and simmer for 5 minutes. Add the remaining ingredients, except for the tomatoes, and continue cooking for 15 minutes over medium heat.

Remove the 4 chunks of squash and puree in a blender. Return the pureed mixture to the pot and let it cook for an additional 10 minutes. Add the tomatoes and cook for another 5 minutes.

Remove from the heat and let sit for 10 minutes to allow the stew to thicken.

Smothered Greens

Cook time: 20–30 minutes   **Yield:** 5 servings

3	cups water
¼	pound skinless smoked turkey breast
1	tablespoon chopped fresh hot pepper
¼	teaspoon cayenne pepper
¼	teaspoon ground cloves
2	cloves garlic, crushed
½	teaspoon thyme
1	scallion, chopped
1	teaspoon ground ginger
¼	cup chopped onion
2	pounds greens (mustard, turnip, collard, kale, or mixture)

Place all ingredients except the greens into a large saucepan and bring to a boil.

Prepare the greens by washing them thoroughly and removing the stems. Tear or slice the leaves into bite-size pieces.

Add the greens to the turkey stock. Cook for 20 to 30 minutes or until tender.

Candied Yams

Cook Time: 20 minutes   **Yield:** 6 servings

- 3 medium yams
- ¼ cup packed brown sugar
- 1 teaspoon flour, sifted
- ¼ teaspoon salt
- ¼ teaspoon ground cinnamon
- ¼ teaspoon ground nutmeg
- ¼ teaspoon grated orange peel
- 1 teaspoon soft tub margarine
- ½ cup orange juice

Preheat the over to 350°F.

Cut the yams in half and boil until tender but firm (about 20 minutes). When cool enough to handle, peel and slice into ¼" thickness.

In a medium bowl, combine the brown sugar, flour, salt, cinnamon, nutmeg, and grated orange peel.

Place half of the sliced yams in a medium casserole dish. Sprinkle with the spiced-sugar mixture. Dot with half the margarine. Add a second layer of yams, using the rest of the ingredients in the order above. Add the orange juice.

Bake uncovered for 20 minutes.

Good-for-You Cornbread

Cook time: 20–25 minutes   **Yield:** 10 servings

- 1   cup cornmeal
- 1   cup flour
- ¼   cup sugar
- 1   teaspoon baking powder
- 1   cup low-fat (1%) buttermilk
- 1   whole egg
- ¼   cup regular tub margarine
- 1   teaspoon vegetable oil

Preheat the oven to 350°F.

In a medium bowl, mix together the cornmeal, flour, sugar, and baking powder.

In a separate small bowl, combine the buttermilk and egg. Beat lightly.

Slowly add the buttermilk and egg mixture to the dry ingredients. Add the margarine and mix by hand or with a mixer for 1 minute.

Bake for 20 to 25 minutes in an 8" x 8", greased baking dish. Cool. Cut into 10 squares.

Savory Potato Salad

Cook time: 25–30 minutes   **Yield:** 10 servings

6	medium potatoes (about 2 pounds)
6	tablespoons mayonnaise
1	teaspoon mustard
½	teaspoon salt
¼	teaspoon black pepper
¼	teaspoon dried dill weed
2	stalks celery, finely chopped
2	scallions, finely chopped
¼	cup coarsely chopped red bell pepper
¼	cup coarsely chopped green bell pepper
1	tablespoon finely chopped onion
1	egg, hard boiled, chopped

Wash the potatoes, cut them in half, and place them in a saucepan of cold water. Cook covered over medium heat for 25 to 30 minutes or until tender. Drain and dice the potatoes once cool.

In a small bowl blend together the mayonnaise, mustard, salt, pepper, and dill weed.

In a big bowl add the vegetables and egg to the potatoes and toss. Pour the dressing over the potato mixture and stir gently to coat evenly.

Chill for at least 1 hour before serving.

Limas and Spinach

Cook time: 15 minutes   **Yield:** 4 servings

2	cups frozen lima beans
½	cup chopped onion
1	cup fennel, cut in 4" strips
1	tablespoon vegetable oil
¼	cup low-sodium chicken broth
4	cups leaf spinach, washed thoroughly
1	tablespoon distilled vinegar
⅙	teaspoon black pepper
1	tablespoon raw chives

Steam or boil the lima beans in unsalted water for about 10 minutes. Drain.

In a medium skillet, cook the onions and fennel in oil. Add the beans and broth to the onions and cover. Cook for 2 minutes. Stir in the spinach. Cover and cook until the spinach has wilted, about 2 minutes. Stir in the vinegar and pepper. Cover and let stand for 30 seconds. Sprinkle with the chives and serve.

Autumn Salad

Cook time: 0 minutes   **Yield:** 6 servings

- 2   tablespoons lemon juice
- 1   medium Granny Smith apple, sliced thin (with skin)
- 1   bag (about 5 cups) mixed lettuce greens (or your favorite lettuce)
- ½   cup dried cranberries
- ¼   cup chopped walnuts
- ¼   cup unsalted sunflower seeds
- ⅓   cup low-fat raspberry vinaigrette dressing

Sprinkle the lemon juice on the apple slices. In a big bowl mix the lettuce, cranberries, apple, walnuts, and sunflower seeds. Toss with the dressing to lightly cover the salad.

Caribbean Casserole

Cook time: 10 minutes   **Yield:** 10 servings

1	medium onion, chopped
½	green bell pepper, diced
1	tablespoon canola oil
1	14.5-ounce can stewed tomatoes
1	16-ounce can black beans (or beans of your choice)
1	teaspoon oregano leaves
½	teaspoon garlic powder
1½	cups instant brown rice, uncooked

In a large pan, cook the onion and green pepper in canola oil, until tender. Do not brown. Add the tomatoes, beans (include the liquid from the broth), oregano, and garlic powder. Bring to a boil. Stir in the rice and cover. Reduce the heat to simmer for 5 minutes. Remove from the heat and let stand for 5 minutes.

Desserts

Mock Southern Sweet Potato Pie

Cook Time: 1 hour   **Yield:** 16 servings

- ¼ cup white sugar
- ¼ cup brown sugar
- ½ teaspoon salt
- ¼ teaspoon nutmeg
- 3 large eggs, beaten
- ¼ cup fat-free evaporated milk
- 1 teaspoon vanilla extract
- 3 cups sweet potatoes (cooked and mashed)

Crust

- 1¼ cups flour
- ¼ teaspoon sugar
- ⅓ cup milk
- 2 tablespoons vegetable oil

Preheat the oven to 350°F.

To make the crust: Combine the flour and sugar in a medium bowl. Add the milk and oil to the flour mixture. Stir with a fork until well mixed. Form the pastry into a smooth ball with your hands. Roll the ball between two 12" squares of wax paper, using short, brisk strokes, until the pastry reaches the edges of the paper. Peel off the top paper and invert the crust into a pie plate.

To make the filling: Combine the sugars, salt, nutmeg, and eggs. Mix in the milk and vanilla. Add the sweet potatoes and mix well. Pour the mixture into the pie shell.

Bake for 1 hour or until the crust is golden brown. Cool and cut into 16 slices.

1-2-3 Peach Cobbler

Cook time: 20–30 minutes   **Yield:** 8 servings

½   teaspoon ground cinnamon
1   tablespoon vanilla extract
2   tablespoons cornstarch
1   cup peach nectar
¼   cup pineapple or peach juice (if desired, use juice reserved from canned peaches)
2   16-ounce cans of peaches, packed in juice (or 1¾ pounds fresh peaches, sliced)
1   tablespoon tub margarine
1   cup dry pancake mix
⅔   cup all-purpose flour
½   cup sugar
⅔   cup fat-free evaporated milk
½   teaspoon nutmeg
1   tablespoon brown sugar
     Nonstick cooking spray, as needed

Preheat the oven to 400°F. Combine the cinnamon, vanilla, cornstarch, peach nectar, and juice in a saucepan over medium heat. Stir constantly until the mixture thickens and bubbles. Add in the sliced peaches. Reduce the heat and simmer for 5 to 10 minutes.

In another saucepan, melt the margarine and set aside.

Lightly spray an 8"-square glass dish with cooking spray. Pour the hot peach mixture into the dish.

In another bowl, combine the pancake mix, flour, sugar, and melted margarine. Stir in the milk. Quickly spoon this mixture over the peach mixture.

In a small bowl combine the nutmeg and brown sugar. Sprinkle the mixture on top of the batter.

Bake for 15 to 20 minutes or until golden brown. Cool and cut into 8 squares.

Southern Banana Pudding

Cook time: 0 minutes   **Yield:** 10 servings

- 3¾ cups cold, fat-free milk
- 2   small packages (4-serving size) fat-free, sugar-free instant vanilla pudding and pie-filling mix
- 32 reduced-fat vanilla wafers
- 2   medium bananas, sliced
- 2   cups fat-free, frozen whipped topping, thawed

In a large bowl, mix 3½ cups of the milk with the pudding mixes. Beat the pudding mixture with a wire whisk for 2 minutes until it is well blended. Let stand for 5 minutes. Fold 1 cup of the whipped topping into the pudding mix.

Arrange a layer of wafers on the bottom and sides of a 2-quart serving bowl. Drizzle 2 tablespoons of the remaining milk over the wafers. Add a layer of banana slices and top with one-third of the pudding.

Repeat the layers, drizzling a wafer layer with the remaining milk and ending with the pudding. Spread the remaining whipped topping over the pudding.

Refrigerate for at least 3 hours before serving.

Resources

THERE ARE MANY FREE SOURCES OF information about diet and exercise activity available for public use. Be aware that when you come across information on the Internet, on TV, in a magazine, or in a promotional pamphlet about these topics, you should first consider where it came from—who provided it, whether the source is credible and/or biased (looking at who funded a brochure or Web site can be telling!), and whether it's consistent with your needs (guidelines for athletes may not be what you're looking for).

However, credible information *does* exist. Below is a list of organizations, Web sites, and books that I trust. Use these to start making smart, educated choices.

The American College of Sports Medicine—a leading fitness organization. acsm.org

The American Diabetes Association—provides information on nutrition, recipes, weight loss, exercise, community programs, local events, and more. diabetes.org

The America Heart Association's Web site contains facts, recipes, and helpful tips for shopping, cooking, and eating out. deliciousdecisions.org

The Centers for Disease Control and Prevention offers solid, reliable information, particularly on exercise guidelines. cdc.gov/physicalactivity/everyone/guidelines/index.html

The Food and Drug Administration provides consumers with warnings and information about federally approved food and drugs in the United States. fda.gov

The U.S. Department of Health and Human Services is a free guide to consumer health information from more than 1,700 health-related government agencies and not-for-profit organizations. healthfinder.gov

Healthy Parks, Healthy People is a national movement that harnesses the power of parks and public lands in contributing to the health and well-being of humans and animals, and the planet we share. nps.gov/public_health/hp/hphp.htm

Let's Move! is a comprehensive initiative launched by Michelle Obama, dedicated to solving the problem of childhood obesity, focusing on solutions so that children born today will grow up healthier and be able to pursue their dreams. letsmove.gov/learn-facts/epidemic-childhood-obesity

The National Heart, Lung, and Blood Institute provides leadership for research, training, and education to promote the prevention and treatment of heart, lung, and blood diseases, and enhance the health of all individuals so that they can live longer and more fulfilling lives. nhlbi.nih.gov

The President's Challenge is a national campaign that encourages all Americans to make being active part of their everyday lives. presidentschallenge.org

The Robert Wood Johnson Foundation focuses on bridging the gap between the nation's health and health care issues. RWJF is currently the country's largest philanthropy devoted exclusively to health and health care. rwjf.org

The Office of Women's Health–Bodyworks, a how-to guide designed to help parents and caregivers of teens and preteens improve family eating and activity habits. womenshealth.gov/bodyworks

The Shriver Report examines the rates of financial insecurity among American women and children, investigates the impact of financial issues on our nation's institutions and economic future, and promotes modern solutions to help women strengthen their financial status. shriverreport.org

Weight Watchers provides recipes and information about eating right and maintaining a healthy lifestyle. weightwatchers.com

The United States Department of Agriculture provides nationally approved dietary guidelines for creating healthy meals every day. choosemyplate.gov

Oprah and Deepak 21-Day Meditation Experience offers insight into the extraordinary power of meditation. chopracentermeditation.com

The Art of Doing Good: Where Passion Meets Action by Charles Bronfman and Jeffrey Solomon is a great book is for anyone setting out to make a difference.

The Book of Awakening by Mark Nepo is a wonderful book about having the life you want by being present in the life you have.

Don't Sweat the Small Stuff by Richard Carlson, PhD, is simple and easy reading for ways to avoid letting the little things take over your life.